16 Super Biohacks
for Longevity

Shortcuts to a Healthier, Happier, Longer Life

Robert Keith Wallace, PhD, Ted Wallace, MS, Samantha Wallace

ISBN 978-1-7357401-5-7

Library of Congress Control Number 2023907139

DharmaPublications.com

Dharma Publications, Fairfield, IA

To Our Very Dear Children and Grandchildren

Gut Crisis
How Diet, Probiotics, and Friendly Bacteria
Help You Lose Weight and Heal Your Body and Mind
Robert Keith Wallace, PhD, Samantha Wallace

Dharma Parenting
Understand Your Child's Brilliant Brain
for Greater Happiness, Health, Success, and Fulfillment
Robert Keith Wallace, PhD, Frederick Travis, PhD

Quantum Golf
The Path to Golf Mastery
REVISED Second Edition
Kjell Enhager, Robert Keith Wallace, PhD, Samantha Wallace

An Introduction to Transcendental Meditation
Improve Your Brain Functioning, Create Ideal Health,
and Gain Enlightenment Naturally, Easily, Effortlessly
Robert Keith Wallace, PhD, Lincoln Akin Norton

Transcendental Meditation
A Scientist's Journey to Happiness, Health, and Peace
Robert Keith Wallace, PhD

The Neurophysiology of Enlightenment
How the Transcendental Meditation and TM-Sidhi Program
Transform the Functioning of the Human Body
Robert Keith Wallace, PhD

Maharishi Ayurveda and Vedic Technology
Creating Ideal Health for the Individual and World
Robert Keith Wallace, PhD

The Coherence Effect
Tapping into the Laws of Nature that Govern Health,
Happiness, and Higher Brain Functioning
Robert Keith Wallace, PhD, Jay B. Marcus,
Christopher S. Clark, MD

CONTENTS

INTRODUCTION

Biohacking and Aging

Will science save us by discovering an innovative technology to extend our life? Some people are betting on it but are not willing to wait for the research. They want to start now, advocating new anti-aging programs. Such approaches are often called *biohacking*, a term first introduced by Dave Asprey, an American entrepreneur who authored the book, *The Bulletproof Diet*. Biohacking involves specific DIY practices to upgrade and protect our health and increase our lifespan ranging from intermittent fasting to meditation, some of these practices are old and some are new, some are free while others are exorbitantly priced.

We live in a world with many health advantages, but it is also a world in which the rise of dementia is alarming. One out of three seniors dies with Alzheimer's or other forms of dementia. Prevention is key and biohacking is becoming increasingly popular among young and old. Scientific research clearly states that the health of the brain follows the simple principle, "Use it or lose it." It's never too late to learn a new language or musical instrument, or, more importantly, a new healthy habit.

Let's start you on the road to biohacking with an easy ancient habit from both Ayurveda and Traditional Chinese Medicine: sip hot or warm water throughout the day. Boil some water, and if you aren't at home put it in a thermos and take it with you. Every few hours take a sip. Almost too easy isn't it? This time-tested tradition is known by ancient medicine to be a powerful detox, and modern medicine agrees that this simple act offers numerous potential benefits, such as increased hydration, thinning excess mucus, and improving circulation. Welcome, you are now biohacking your longevity and at no cost.

Aging

Why do we age in the first place? Everything is working perfectly and then we are surprised when our health begins to slide downhill. Scientists have attempted to explain aging with many single dominant theories, such as programmed longevity, free radical theory, or the membrane theory of aging. The membrane theory, for example, says that cells are impaired because age related changes affect the cell membrane's chemicals and electrical processes. These are interesting ideas backed by valid research findings, but most would agree that they are incomplete.

Aging is the result of a combination of many factors that can be summarized by the expression "nature versus nurture," which means we are born with a certain DNA, and then everything we do has an impact on our health and aging. Most researchers consider that our individual genetic heritage accounts for about 20–40% of our chance to live a longer life. The Ashkenazi Jews seem to have won the longevity genes sweepstakes. Even though some of them smoke and have other unhealthy habits, they can still live to over 95 in a healthy state. For the rest of us, our longevity depends a great deal on the way we live our lives from childhood onward.

The science of epigenetics studies how environmental factors affect the expression of genes in our DNA; causing some specific genes to be turned on, while others are turned off. Every action, from the foods we eat to our daily exercise, affects gene expression and ultimately determines our health and lifespan.

Modern Biohacks

Some biohacking ideas are extremely experimental, such as getting a transfusion of "young blood." Young blood has been studied in animals and refers to transferring the blood from younger animals to an older animal to improve their health. The technical name for this procedure is *parabiosis* in which the circulatory system of one animal is connected to that of another. When an older animal is connected to a younger animal, the older animals begin to exhibit rejuvenation in certain tissues such as the skeletal muscles, heart, and liver, and even show improvements in memory. In contrast, the younger animal experiences an opposite effect. Their tissues age more quickly , and they demonstrate a loss in memory.

The main conclusion from this and other research is that blood from young animals seems to restore youthful gene expression patterns in certain tissues, while blood from biologically older animals has the opposite effect. Clearly, there are rejuvenating factors in young blood, and aging factors in the blood from the older animals. Can we make an animal live longer through infusions of young blood? Present research does not bear this idea out. If we are not able to extend the life of an entire animal, can we at least use this method to rejuvenate certain tissues in humans?

As is often the case, the findings in animals do not always apply to humans and to even study blood transfusion in humans involves many comprehensive levels of approval. Instead attempts have been made to isolate the rejuvenating factors. One of the most well documented is a factor called growth differentiation factor named GDF11 peptide. Researchers at Harvard claimed that GDF11 levels in blood fell with age, and that supplementing GDF11 could revitalize old muscles including heart muscles. These studies, however, have had conflicting results. Other scientists are searching for how to use precursors of GDF11 or other more promising rejuvenating factors.

New experimental biohacks for longevity need to be researched thoroughly to make sure that there are no adverse side effects, like those exhibited in so many modern pharmaceuticals. Despite the lack of concrete evidence, companies are already competing to monetize these new findings. This comes with obvious ethical concerns. One start-up company began selling young blood plasma transfusions for $8,000 per liter.

Ancient Biohacks

There are many effective ancient biohacks. The focus of my own research over the last 50 years has been on meditation and Ayurveda, specifically Transcendental Meditation and Maharishi AyurVeda, which are both from the ancient Vedic tradition of India. Is it alright to call the profound and time-tested techniques of this tradition by the name biohacks? To some it might seem inappropriate, but it is the language of modern times, and it is important to convey this valuable knowledge in a way that will be more easily understood.

The ancient science of Ayurveda is the natural health system of India and has innumerable recommendations to prevent and treat disease. It also offers herbal supplements and special treatments that focus on longevity. Some Ayurveda biohacks benefit everyone, like the advice to have our main meal at noon when digestion is the strongest. Other biohacks depend upon our individual mind/body nature and are highly personalized. Ayurveda describes three main mind/body natures or Energy States, called Vata, Pitta, and Kapha.

For a Vata individual the most effective biohack is to stick to a daily routine. For a Pitta person the most important biohack is to not miss a meal. The word "hangry" was surely coined for them. Finally, for the Kapha Energy State people, a good biohack is to keep active. Each of us is a mixture of these three Energy States, and the best biohacks for each will most likely include a blend of different behaviors and food. Throughout this book we will discuss many valuable biohacks from Ayurveda.

BIOHACK #1

THE SECRET OF BIOHACKING

The secret of biohacking is the ability to turn a biohack into a habit. Your biohacks will only increase your lifespan when they become an integral part of your life. "The ultimate purpose of habits is to solve the problems of life with as little energy and effort as possible," says James Clear, author of the bestselling book *Atomic Habits*. Clear suggests four laws of change: 1) make it obvious, 2) make it attractive, 3) make it easy, and 4) make it satisfying. Most of us decide to improve our lives by making a list of firm resolutions, which we forget about in a month or a week.

Simple Habits

It can help enormously to keep the habit as simple as possible by only making one small change at a time. This is exactly what James Clear suggests: "An atomic habit is a little habit that is part of a larger system. Just as atoms are the building blocks of molecules, atomic habits are the building blocks of remarkable results."

Many other habit change experts agree, including B.J. Fogg,

author of *Tiny Habits*. Start small and build over time. Before you know it, your life will be reshaped by your new habits. James Clear goes on to say, "Ultimately, your habits matter because they help you become the type of person you wish to be. They are the channel through which you develop your deepest beliefs about yourself. Quite literally, you become your habits." This very interesting concept suggests that our habits are far more important than we may have thought.

Ayurveda and Habit Change

Ayurveda also emphasizes starting with one small doable habit. But it adds a whole new perspective to habit change. Why is it so easy for some people to transform a biohack into a habit while for others it's hard? We are all different and the sooner we discover who we are, the sooner we can improve our lives. Ayurveda and many other systems of traditional health have a procedure for understanding what is best for each of us. They personalize health and learning. Let's take a simple quiz to find out who we are according to Ayurveda. This will give valuable insight into how we can more easily transform our biohacks into habits.

Energy State Quiz

V Energy State	*Strongly Disagree / Strongly Agree*				
1. Light sleeper, difficulty falling asleep	[1]	[2]	[3]	[4]	[5]
2. Irregular appetite	[1]	[2]	[3]	[4]	[5]
3. Learns quickly but forgets quickly	[1]	[2]	[3]	[4]	[5]
4. Easily becomes overstimulated	[1]	[2]	[3]	[4]	[5]
5. Does not tolerate cold weather very well	[1]	[2]	[3]	[4]	[5]
6. A sprinter rather than a marathoner	[1]	[2]	[3]	[4]	[5]
7. Speech is energetic, with frequent changes in topic	[1]	[2]	[3]	[4]	[5]
8. Anxious and worried when under stress	[1]	[2]	[3]	[4]	[5]
V Score	*(Total your responses)*				

P ENERGY STATE	STRONGLY DISAGREE / STRONGLY AGREE				
1. Easily becomes overheated	[1]	[2]	[3]	[4]	[5]
2. Strong reaction when challenged	[1]	[2]	[3]	[4]	[5]
3. Uncomfortable when meals are delayed	[1]	[2]	[3]	[4]	[5]
4. Good at physical activity	[1]	[2]	[3]	[4]	[5]
5. Strong appetite	[1]	[2]	[3]	[4]	[5]
6. Good sleeper but may not need as much sleep as others	[1]	[2]	[3]	[4]	[5]
7. Clear and precise speech	[1]	[2]	[3]	[4]	[5]
8. Becomes irritable and/or angry under stress	[1]	[2]	[3]	[4]	[5]
P SCORE	(TOTAL YOUR RESPONSES)				

K ENERGY STATE	STRONGLY DISAGREE / STRONGLY AGREE				
1. Slow eater	[1]	[2]	[3]	[4]	[5]
2. Falls asleep easily but wakes up slowly	[1]	[2]	[3]	[4]	[5]
3. Steady, stable temperament	[1]	[2]	[3]	[4]	[5]
4. Doesn't mind waiting to eat	[1]	[2]	[3]	[4]	[5]
5. Slow to learn but rarely forgets	[1]	[2]	[3]	[4]	[5]
6. Good physical strength and stamina	[1]	[2]	[3]	[4]	[5]
7. Speech may be slow and thoughtful	[1]	[2]	[3]	[4]	[5]
8. Possessive and stubborn under stress	[1]	[2]	[3]	[4]	[5]
K SCORE	(TOTAL YOUR RESPONSES)				

Compare all three scores. Whichever total is higher, V, P, or K, is your primary Energy State. It is common to have two high scores and one lower score. This shows that you are a combination of two main Energy States, with a minor influence from the third. In some cases, you may have three similar scores. This is somewhat rare and indicates that you are a Tri-Energy State. You may also find that your score highlights only one Energy State. This means that every aspect of your life is strongly influenced by this Energy State.

Energy States

Individuals with a predominant V Energy State tend to be creative, curious, and enthusiastic. They are your inventive, artistic friends. In business, they can produce innovative customer oriented marketing campaigns.

Individuals with a P Energy State are purposeful and dynamic achievers and are often competitive athletic partners or adversaries. In business, they are frequently goal-oriented leaders of teams and companies.

People who have a K Energy State are often very stable, relaxed, and good-natured. These are the steady, grounded friends who help you through challenging times, and in business they frequently hold the position of trustworthy administrators; they are good at increasing harmony and cooperation.

Habit Change and Energy State

Each Energy State shows a different tendency toward learning a new habit. V Energy State people are quick to learn but they may have a hard time sticking to a new habit. The attention of a V Energy State person can be very precise but also tends to move rapidly from one topic to another. They are sensitive and can be overwhelmed by too many choices. Pushing a V individual to learn a new habit can result in a strong reaction. And if this reaction becomes overly emotional and out of balance, it will be almost impossible for them to focus their attention on habit change until they are again balanced and calm.

Adopting a new habit is relatively easy for P Energy State people. They are primarily interested in solutions and in achieving goals. Many habit change books seem to be written by P Energy State individuals for P Energy State individuals.

K Energy State people have a harder time making a new change and can be extremely attached to a routine. They like to think things through thoroughly and methodically before making decisions. They will be better able to execute a habit change when they have some support from a partner or friend.

Neurohacking the Learning Cycle

Neurohacking is a lot like biohacking, except its focus is on the brain. Neurohacking the learning cycle means figuring out how to adopt a habit more quickly and efficiently. There are 4 main components to the learning cycle: motivate, personalize, experiment, and be real.

Motivation is everything. It is hard to learn a new habit if you are not motivated. Motivation can come from fear or inspiration. You could be afraid of getting sick and dying young, and therefore be willing to exercise more. Or, you could be determined to be healthy and fit and thus be inspired to exercise. Motivation is easier if you have a clear intention. Some intentions are simple and concrete, others are abstract and all-encompassing. Both are valuable, but habits are generally easier to learn if they are tied to your sense of identity, of who you want to become in your life.

Personalize your habits. Each of us needs a different approach to habit change. Ayurveda makes this very clear. If you are a P Energy State person it's much easier to adopt new habits, but what about others who are not as driven? They need to create strategies that will help them adopt a new habit according to who they are.

Experiment with different biohacks until you decide on the ones that you want to make a permanent habit. We teach a simple method of creating a Habit Map and Plan so you can be more effective in experimenting.

Be real is a phrase that reminds us that when we transform a biohack into a habit we need constant feedback. Are we exercising regularly? Are there obstacles that are holding us back? Are we making our best effort?

Here's an example of how to use these 4 components for adopting a habit.

Adopting a New Habit

Motivate

Begin by writing a sentence about something you want to change in your life. Do you want to drink more water? Do you want to become a writer or an artist? It's alright to start with a big idea if you understand that what you are trying to do is create a series of small habits to achieve that bigger goal. Place this statement in the center of a piece of paper or on your computer screen as the beginning your Habit Map. For example, "I want to lose 15 pounds over the next three months."

Personalize

Make it personal. You understand that you are part Pitta and part Kapha so you have to find a small habit that will help you achieve this goal. Around your central goal, in the center of your Habit Map, like spokes radiating from the hub of a wheel, list some small simple habits that you believe you can do. Taking a 15 minute walk each day could be one idea. Eating fewer calories is another. Maybe eating more slowly and putting more attention on your food would help. Remember, you are part Kapha so your metabolism is a little slower than others and you can gain weight easily. You are also part Pitta and tend to eat quickly and may not pay enough attention to the quantity and quality of the food you are eating.

Experiment

Now comes the fun part. Out of all your ideas on the spokes of your Habit Map, pick one small, specific habit that appeals to you such as, "I am going to eat more slowly and pay more attention to how I am eating the food. I will help myself do this by lowering my fork between each bite of food. I will try this for a month and see how it affects my weight and how I feel." This is your Habit Plan. Instead of rushing through your meal without really savoring it, this new habit will allow you to both taste and appreciate your food more completely.

Part of the experiment is finding a *cue* or *prompt* that will help you remember to practice this habit. One possible cue might be the act of sitting down and taking your first bite. Another would be to have your partner, a friend, or a family member remind you of this new habit when you sit down. It doesn't have to be a scolding, just a kind reminder in the right direction. You could even have some fun and put a large fork in the center of the table as a cue. Each person needs to find a unique cue that works for them.

Be Real

The fourth component is to be genuinely honest about your progress: *Be Real*. To do this you need feedback. Are you able to adopt the new biohack and make it into a habit? In the book *Total Brain Coaching* we developed a tool called the Feedback Matrix which uses 4 four levels of feedback from: self coaching, personal coaching, group coaching, and environmental coaching.

Self coaching is the first level of feedback, where you maintain a journal or use a journaling app. In your journal, you objectively assess your progress and reflect subjectively on how well you are doing. This may require some extra effort, but it provides a clear record of your progress and valuable insights for improvement.

The second level of feedback comes from personal coaching. It can be helpful to have a buddy who can check in with you and see how you are doing. While it may not always be easy to find someone to assist you, it is important to try. Even if you are a person with strong willpower (P Energy State), having a buddy is a valuable strategy.

You can check in with your buddy at the end of each day or, if that doesn't work, perhaps once a week. The ideal question your buddy can ask is, "Are you doing your best to maintain your habit?" You can rate your efforts on a scale of 1 to 10. It's alright to have setbacks or low scores on certain days due to obstacles or distractions. Discuss these challenges with your buddy, and when things normalize, give it another try.

If possible, working with a professional coach can be ideal as they can help you identify goals and milestones. Coaches typically provide an overview of the coaching sessions and establish a code of conduct. Their role is to help you find solutions, and they often ask, "What do you want to achieve by the end of our 45-minute session today?" Changing a habit often requires time, energy, and sometimes external support.

Group coaching, the third level of feedback, can be conducted in person or online. Working with a group can be highly beneficial as you observe how others cope with the challenges of maintaining new habits. It can be particularly valuable to have participants from different Energy State types, creating an interactive and dynamic environment.

The fourth and final type of feedback is environmental coaching. Although we might think of ourselves as independent from our environment, this is usually not the case. For example, if your new habit is to avoid snacking between meals, you can ask your partner or family for support by removing snacks from your home during that time. Altering your environment can aid in habit change. Experimentation is key—try different ideas until you find what works for you. If nothing seems effective after a month, you can return to the Habit Map and experiment with adopting a new habit.

Finally, there is the aspect of rewards. If you successfully accomplish your goal, it is important to celebrate and reward yourself. It can be as simple as having fun with those who supported you throughout the process. Rewarding yourself enhances motivation and boosts confidence to adopt more habits.

Super Habits

Super Habits are special habits that can help improve life. B.J. Fogg, for example, introduced what he calls the Maui Habit; he suggests that when you get up each day, the moment your feet first touch the floor, you say, "It's going to be a great day." It turns out that daily gratitude is a powerful Super Habit. Before you go to sleep every night, try writing down 3 or 4 things you are grateful for (you can repeat the same things each night). The Super Habit which we highly recommend is meditation, particularly Transcendental Meditation (TM).

BIOHACK #2

MEDITATE

What can you do when you are feeling stressed, tense, haven't had enough sleep, and have had too much coffee? How about a few chocolates to ease the anxiety? Nope, can't do that because your gut is too upset. It's like everything in you is moving too fast, not a moment of relaxation. You check your social media for the latest news: no good, more mass shootings. What about a walk or a massage? Not enough time or cash. Turmoil inside and out, uncomfortable all over.

Heart disease may be listed as the #1 killer today, but underlying heart disease and other physical and mental problems is an overload of stress. And that same stress can cause you to adopt unhealthy habits, like smoking or eating too much, just to feel even a little bit better for a short while. However, these compensatory habits put you at further risk for heart disease. The modern world keeps getting more stressful, so we have to find ways to counteract stress.

Meditation is the natural antidote. You might also take a walk on the beach or in the woods, but meditation is even easier and more powerful. The problem is that most meditation techniques are hard to do; people start them but then stop. Of course, you can get a meditation app and be guided through a session and there may be some calm but is it really countering the damaging effects of stress? Do you enjoy the practice enough to make a habit of meditating regularly? Regularity is what it really takes to manage stress and anxiety.

Different Types of Meditation

My research has focused on the Transcendental Meditation program and it has become clear to me that it is by far the easiest and most effective meditation technique. Volumes of research support it, clearly showing that TM produces a state of restful alertness which counteracts the effects of stress, while improving our ability to adapt to challenging situations. There are so many studies that I will only mention a few here: In one extremely well-controlled clinical trial funded by the National Institutes of Health (NIH) and led by Robert Schneider, MD, there was a 48% reduction in heart attacks, strokes, and deaths in the TM group as compared to controls. Additional studies have shown that TM can reverse the effects of aging and can extend lifespan. It improves creativity and intelligence, and more. It even changes the expression of genes in our DNA.

How is TM different from other techniques? The ancient practices of Zen, Compassion Meditation, Qigong, Diamond Way Buddhism, Zazen, Kriya Yoga, and more recent practices of

Mindfulness and Mindfulness-Based Stress Reduction (MBSR) are different from Transcendental Meditation. Drs. Fred Travis and Jonathan Shear published a paper in which they identified three major categories of "meditation" to compare more than a hundred different practices. These three are summarized as follows:

> *Focused attention*: The first type of practice can be described as concentration meditation, since in this case, the practitioner puts his or her attention intently on something (it might be a word, an emotion, a candle flame, etc.). The changes in the brain electrical activity are seen as activation in the gamma range (20–50 Hz), which is known to be associated with this type of focused activity. Some forms of Zen, Compassion Meditation, Qigong, and Diamond Way Buddhism are in this category.

> *Open monitoring*: The second of type of practice can be described as contemplation meditation. In this process, the practitioner watches himself or herself do something, such as paying attention to thoughts or the breath. This category includes Zazen, Kriya Yoga, and more recently developed versions of meditation like Mindfulness. The changes in the brain from these meditations are shown as electrical activity in the theta range (4–8 Hz), known to be associated with imagination and creativity (and sometimes drowsiness).

> *Automatic self-transcending*: This third type of practice can be described as transcending meditation. In this practice there is no trying, no concentration, and no contemplation—only effortless transcending. The changes in the brain EEG are in the alpha 1 range (8–10 Hz) and are correlated with an eyes-closed, relaxed state of restful alertness. Transcendental Meditation falls into this category.

The TM technique is a unique, simple, and effective mental procedure that is practiced for about twenty minutes, twice each day, sitting comfortably with your eyes closed. It involves no belief or philosophy, no mood or lifestyle. Most people begin the technique for practical reasons, such as a desire for more energy or to decrease tension and anxiety, and over ten million people of all ages, cultures, and religious backgrounds have learned TM. We hear a lot about famous movie stars, business leaders, athletes, musicians, scientists, and talk show hosts who all practice TM. But hundreds of thousands more—homemakers, teachers, veterans, bank clerks, farmers, small business owners, students of all ages, from every imaginable walk of life—are quietly and effortlessly practicing the TM program, benefiting from the release of stress, and increasing their success and happiness at work and at home.

Some people think they can't meditate because their minds are too active; others think they can't do it because it will be too hard. TM uses the nature of the mind to go to fields of greater happiness—to go within. No "trying" is involved. If you try, your mind remains on the surface and cannot dive deep. Transcendence is a real experience that isn't based on a mood or emotion.

The following is a quote from the book *The Coherence Effect* by Jay Marcus, Dr. Chris Clark, and me. It is from a woman who entered West Point in 1976. She graduated, was commissioned as an officer in 1980, served in the military for five years, and then became a nurse. From the moment she entered the Academy, as part of the Academy's first class of women, she experienced severe anxiety. She went through 20 years of therapy, medication, and different stress management techniques until she eventually ly learned TM.

Over almost twenty years I tried all the other meditation techniques: Siddha Yoga, Forest Zen, Japanese Zen, Buddhist and Christian contemplative, mindfulness meditation. TM is the best!

I tried all these other practices and was only partially successful. Some of them worked, but again only partially. With mindfulness I had a lot of trouble with it, and I just didn't find it very helpful. I couldn't actually settle down and relax. It didn't get rid of all the thoughts in my head. It wasn't what I wanted.

TM was different, and it worked from the very beginning. It is much deeper than the other practices and really helps me put my body into a restful state and then at the same time, it clears out my head. I really look forward to the calmness it brings, and I seem to tap into inner resources that I did not know I had. The mood swings that were prevalent in my life are gone. I've acquired a new ability to respond to situations in a healthy way, instead of feeling confused or angry and reacting in that state. My physical health has improved too. I have more vitality, and 50 percent of the chronic pain is gone, and I can recover from illness in days instead of weeks or months. I think this should be a program in every VA Medical Center. I see mindfulness-based meditation courses all the time. But I have tried all these meditation techniques and they just aren't the same as TM.

TM cannot properly be learned from books, it must be taught through the personal instruction from a trained and certified teacher. Correct instruction helps the meditator avoid any trying, straining, or expectation. Effort, according to Maharishi Mahesh

Yogi, who developed and popularized TM, will hold the mind on the gross level and prevent the experience of more delicate and subtle levels of the thinking process.

TM Improves Neuroadaptability

Your brain is incredibly flexible and active. You have probably heard the word *neuroplasticity,* which is used to describe the brain's ability to change even at an older age. Neuroadaptability is a special type of neuroplasticity that refers to the brain's ability to adapt to challenging or threatening situations.

To illustrate how neuroadaptability works, let's look at the brain of someone who just encountered a threat. In such an emergency, your brain typically initiates the "fight or flight response." A small and potent part of the brain called the amygdala becomes activated. The amygdala is the seat of your greatest fears and phobias and is connected to a structure called the hippocampus, which has access to memories and emotions. These two areas are connected to the higher centers in your prefrontal cortex where information is interpreted. Is that a life-threatening snake in front of you…or is it a piece of rope?

If the threat is perceived to be real, the amygdala and hippocampus will act immediately, without waiting for any interpretation from the higher centers in the prefrontal cortex. Signals are sent to the hypothalamus, pituitary gland, and adrenal glands. When the fight or flight response is turned on, our heart beats faster, our blood pressure rises, and we shunt blood away from digestive organs to our muscles. The sympathetic nervous system becomes activated and there is a surge of the neurotransmitter noradrenalin (norepinephrine). There is also the release of the hormone adrenalin (epinephrine) along with the secretion of cortisol, both from the adrenal glands.

The fight or flight response gives us a huge evolutionary advantage when we are being chased by a wild predator. But what happens to our brain and body in chronic stress when this response is repeatedly turned on in situations that do not require it? It can be as simple as being stuck in a traffic jam, or having to endlessly hold the phone as you wait to speak to a human customer service agent. The result of such apparently harmless situations is far from simple—they lead to a constantly elevated level of cortisol which is detrimental to both your physical and mental health.

Unremittingly elevated levels of cortisol can depress your immune system, shut down your digestion, and result in long term gut problems. Over time, high cortisol levels also have negative effects on parts of your brain. The cells in the prefrontal cortex and hippocampus, for example, become damaged and less responsive, while cells in the amygdala become functionally and structurally modified so that they continually overreact to stress. These changes occur on many levels, including neural circuits, receptors in our neural membranes, and the molecular mechanisms that regulate gene expression.

The destruction of cells in the hippocampus is especially debilitating since this area of the brain is critically involved in emotion and memory. You need your hippocampus to be able to compare present and past dangers, and help dampen the stress response, since it helps limit the secretion of cortisol when there is no real threat.

Chronic stress eventually causes or exacerbates other disorders such as high blood pressure, irritable bowel syndrome, anxiety and depression. In the case of high blood pressure, it is as if your internal blood pressure regulator becomes stuck on high, even when the supposed threat no longer exists. Such side effects are only the tip of the stress iceberg. Poor neuroadaptive behavior can also lead to drug, alcohol, and other addictions.

Our environment will always throw challenges at us, but learning TM and improving our neuroadaptability can help us become more flexible and effective. We need to be able to react appropriately to stressful situations, and we also need to return quickly to a normal healthy state. Restful alertness and coherence are the basis of appropriate positive neuroadaptability.

Research on TM

Drs. Harold Harung and Fred Travis have studied the EEG brain wave signature of individuals functioning at the highest level of performance in business, sports, and music. This EEG signature consists of coherent alpha brain waves being produced in the frontal areas of the brain. Alpha waves reveal a relaxed state of awareness, and increased coherence indicates greater integration among different parts of the brain. This EEG pattern is also seen in long term practitioners of TM who have improved levels of neuroadaptability. More importantly, TM research shows that it is possible to reach an optimal state of brain functioning, which results in better physical and mental health.

More than 600 studies at over 200 research institutes and universities have been conducted on the Transcendental Meditation program, and over 380 of these studies have been published in top journals. The US National Institutes of Health has awarded over $25 million in grants to study the effects of TM on health, particularly on heart disease, and a statement from the American Heart Association concluded:

> The Transcendental Meditation technique is the only meditation practice that has been shown to lower blood pressure.
> Because of many negative studies or mixed results and a paucity of available trials, all other meditation techniques (including MBSR) received a 'Class III, no benefit, Level of Evidence C' recommendation. Thus, other meditation techniques are not recommended in clinical practice to lower BP at this time.
> Transcendental Meditation practice is recommended for consideration in treatment plans for all individuals with blood pressure > 120/80 mm Hg. Lower blood pressure through Transcendental Meditation practice is also associated with substantially reduced rates of death, heart attack, and stroke.

Studies have documented how TM can slow and even reverse

the aging process. One early study showed that long-term TM meditators had a biological age which was roughly twelve years younger than their non-meditating counterparts. Another study conducted at Harvard studied the effects of TM on mental health, behavioral flexibility, blood pressure, and longevity in residents of homes for the elderly. The subjects were randomly assigned to either a no-treatment group or one of three treatment programs: the TM program, mindfulness training, or a relaxation program. All three groups were initially similar on pretest measures and in expectancy of benefits, yet after a three-month experimental period, the TM group had significant improvements in cognitive functioning and blood pressure as compared to the control groups. Also, the TM subjects reported deeper experiences during their practice and were feeling better and more relaxed immediately afterward than did the mindfulness or the relaxation subjects. Overall, more TM subjects found their practice to be personally valuable than did members of either of the control groups.

The most striking finding was that TM practice not only reversed age-related declines in overall health, but also directly enhanced longevity. All members of the TM group were still alive three years after the program began, in contrast to about only half of the members of the control groups. Research on the TM technique clearly shows that growing old no longer needs to signify a loss in the quality of life; rather, it can be an opportunity for further development.

Another important study on aging involves the measurement of one of the most reliable biochemical markers of the aging process, serum dehydroepiandrosterone sulfate (DHEAS). DHEAS declines progressively with age. Peak levels occur in one's mid-twenties; by the eighth and ninth decades of life, one's DHEAS level may have declined by 80 percent. The mean DHEAS levels in meditators practicing TM were significantly higher than in the controls. The levels measured in the older meditators were generally comparable to levels in control groups five to ten years younger.

Dr. Robert Schneider and his coworkers have shown in their studies on cardiovascular disease that TM improves health and promotes longer life. In one longitudinal study TM subjects showed an increased telomere length, again suggesting a reversal of the aging process. Telomeres are a part of the DNA which are found at the end of chromosomes. They maintain the integrity of the chromosome and normally shorten with cell division as we get older.

The results of these studies strongly indicate that the TM program slows the aging process. Two distinct types of underlying physiological mechanisms that might account for these long-term changes are: (1) an increased ability to maintain a lower, more stable, internal resting state, and (2) an improved, more adaptable response to external stress. For more information about TM, go to TM.org. where you can find links to studies and other useful information.

From Biohack to Habit

Let's say you decide to learn the ultimate biohack, Transcendental Meditation. How can you make this biohack into a habit so that you can comfortably practice it for 20 minutes twice a day? If you learned TM from a qualified instructor there will already be many clear guidelines to make sure you are doing it correctly and effortlessly. And there is a built-in reward because you are probably noticing improvements in your life. And with your new-found energy and creativity you start to be even more productive. It's time to apply the tools we learned from Neurohacking the Learning Cycle.

Motivation is not a problem because TM is easy, and you are getting good results. The technique is personalized, and it works equally well for each of the different Energy States. What about experiment? If you want to be regular in your practice, then it is useful to experiment with things that will make it easier for you to be more consistent.

Your intention is simple, "I want to be more consistent with my TM practice." That goes in a circle in the center of the plan. Now add other ideas around this main idea. You can put the online group meditation as the first one. Next, you might add a reminder on your phone that notifies you when it is time to start your meditation. You might decide to meditate with your partner or a friend to keep you on track. Pick any one of these, and then choose a cue and a reward. Be real and find out if your experiment really works. To complete your Biohack Map and Plan follow the steps below using the graphic.

Step 1: Enter your main intention or desire for your biohack in the center.

Step 2: Around the central idea for the biohack enter some action steps that you think will help accomplish your change.

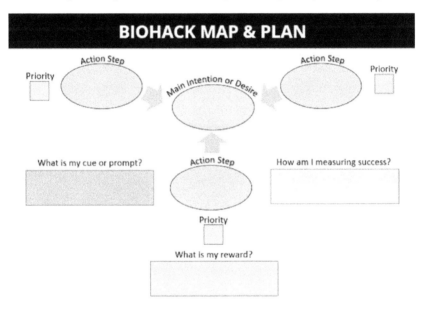

Step 3: Prioritize your list and choose the main action step that you want to use.

Step 4: Enter a cue or prompt that will help you remember to do your new action step.

Step 5: Determine how you will measure your success with the new biohack and create a reward.

Step 6: Use feedback from self coaching, personal coaching, group coaching, and environmental coaching to keep improving your ability to adopt new habits.

BIOHACK #3

MORNING SUNLIGHT

Can something as simple as walking in the beautiful golden rays of the early morning sun produce measurable health benefits? Although I had heard this recommendation from one of the greatest experts in Ayurveda, I had no idea how the mechanics of the physiology were involved until new research suggested how this seemingly simple biohack might work.

First, what is sunlight? Second, how does it affect our body and mind? Third, what chemicals are affected by light which have positive effects on the body?

Sunlight

Why is the sky blue at noon, but golden red at sunrise and sunset? The light from the sun is a combination of visible light, ultraviolet light, and infrared light. The visible light from the sun is white light, which is made up of all the colors of the rainbow. Clouds are white because they contain droplets of water which reflect all the colors to produce white. At noon, we mostly see a blue sky, because blue wavelengths of light are short, just the right size to be scattered by air molecules in the atmosphere. Blue light is everywhere in the sky and dominates our vision.

At sunrise, when the sun is low in the sky, the rays of light must travel farther through more of the atmosphere before we can see them. The blue and other shorter wavelengths are scattered away from our vision so the red and yellow rays are more obvious.

The light at sunrise also has infrared and near infrared (NIR) light rays that we can't see but that have a big effect on our body. There are studies that show the many beneficial effects of the right dose of infrared light, and it is now used in several types of therapy. Certainly, too much bright sunlight can be bad for our skin, causing UV damage and even skin cancer. Please note we are not advocating an entire day in the sun, just a few minutes at and around sunrise.

The Beneficial Effects of Light

Vitamin D, of course, is produced by the interaction of sunlight with our skin and has many beneficial effects in the body. How else does sunlight affect us? One of most important effects is that it puts us in sync with the natural rhythms of nature. The light from the sun stimulates a newly discovered pigment in our eyes known as melanopsin. Melanopsin is produced by special cells in the eye known as intrinsically photosensitive retinal ganglion cells. Unlike the rods and cones in our retina, these cells are not concerned with vision, but rather with non-vision-related functions of light, most importantly for resetting biological rhythms. The activation of melanopsin leads to signals being sent to various parts of your brain. The primary effect is to stimulate the central biological clock in the suprachiasmatic nucleus of your hypothalamus. Light synchronizes the clock to be in tune with nature's 24-hour or circadian rhythm and allows it to reset all the many different clocks in the cells of your body. This is important since being out of tune with the natural daily circadian rhythms increases the risk for many diseases. Signals are then sent from the hypothalamus to the pineal gland and other areas of the body causing a turning-off of the production of melatonin, the sleep hormone, and a turning-on of cortisol, the waking hormone. We normally think of cortisol as a stress hormone, but your body requires a certain level of cortisol to function normally.

What other effects come from morning sunlight? It contains red light, and we know that red light therapy, which is also known as low-level light therapy (LLLT) and photobiomodulation (PBM therapy), has shown many positive effects. Red (630 to 660 nm) and near infrared (NIR) (810 to 850 nm) light can increase ATP production in our mitochondria, stimulate cerebral blood flow, cause the regrowth of neurons (a process called neurogenesis), and positively affect certain neurological and psychiatric disorders.

Dr. Mohammad Muneeb Khan, an oncologist in England, has suggested that early morning sunlight penetrates our skin and stimulates the production of melatonin from the mitochondria. The mitochondria are the powerplants in virtually every cell of our body. They even have their own DNA which is different from the DNA in the cell nucleus. The melatonin produced in the mitochondria is independent of the melatonin produced by the pineal gland. More importantly, it has been shown to be an extremely powerful antioxidant with various healing properties.

Sunlight a great example of an easy biohack! Get up in the morning, take a walk, and experience the light of the sun. It is totally enjoyable and has many side-benefits. A sunrise walk has been, and still is, recommended by the oldest and greatest traditions of natural medicine. We have to wonder how many other ancient biohacks will become modern scientific rediscoveries that allow us to live healthier, happier, and longer lives! Time and more research will tell.

From Biohack to Habit

Let's say you want to take an early morning walk every day. How can you make this biohack a habit? To complete your Biohack Map and Plan follow the steps below using the graphic.

Step 1: Enter your main intention or desire for your biohack in the center.

Step 2: Around the central idea for the biohack enter some action steps that you think will help accomplish your change.

Step 3: Prioritize your list and choose the main action step that you want to use.

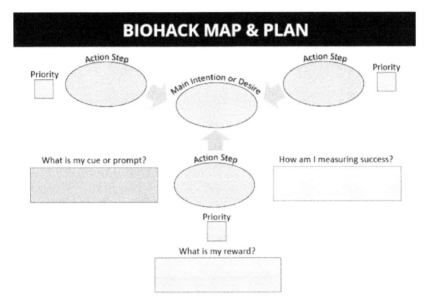

Step 4: Enter a cue or prompt that will help you remember to do your new action step.

Step 5: Determine how you will measure your success with the new biohack and create a reward.

Step 6: Use feedback from self coaching, personal coaching, group coaching, and environmental coaching to keep improving your ability to adopt new habits.

BIOHACK #4

EAT LESS

So far, the most conclusive research that shows an extension of the lifespan in animals does so by reducing their caloric intake. Hundreds of studies have shown that by reducing the number of calories an animal regularly eats, they live longer. Very few studies, however, have been done on humans for the simple reason that it is hard to get subjects to voluntarily reduce their food intake over a long period of time. The eminent Harvard geneticist David Sinclair expressed the problem very clearly: "I tried calorie restriction and couldn't do it. It's really hard to be hungry all the time."

In his best-selling book *Lifespan*, Sinclair goes deeply into how caloric reduction might work. He identifies several survival pathways and genes which he believes are crucial to maintaining health and extending life. Caloric restriction acts as an epigenetic challenge, which causes certain genes to be affected. The most important anti-aging genes are the 7 sirtuin genes and signaling proteins (SIRT1–SIRT7) that enable different processes that could extend life—including DNA repair, stress resistance, and reduction of inflammation. Sinclair also discusses specific supplements which he feels can modify these pathways.

Anti-Aging Pathways

One longevity supplement, called nicotinamide adenine dinucleotide or NAD, is known to energize the sirtuin pathway and, in fact, boost the activity of all 7 sirtuin proteins. Another supplement, resveratrol, derived from grape skins, is used to stimulate the SIRT1 protein. Since resveratrol is present in wine, experts have used it to explain the so-called "French Paradox," the phenomenon in France where there are lower rates of heart attacks despite the high consumption of saturated fats in butter and meat. Studies on animals have shown that the combination of resveratrol and caloric restriction can markedly extend lifespan. But resveratrol, like many other anti-aging substances, isn't assimilated very well by our body. To have a positive effect, you would have to use a higher dose, the equivalent of consuming many bottles of wine per day. It is also unclear if resveratrol can directly activate sirtuins when taken orally. Research goes on to look for better anti-aging substances.

One other possibility is quercetin, which is a plant flavonoid found in many fruits and vegetables. Quercetin has many potential uses. The word "quercetin" is derived from the Latin word *quercetum* which means oak forest. Quercetin has been observed to increase SIRT1 activity fivefold, and it has been found to act as a senolytic, a compound that can eliminate old senescent cells. Again, however, quercetin's therapeutic value is limited in humans by its inability to reach the appropriate tissues.

Quercetin and other supplements have been found to act on

another longevity pathway, the mammalian target of rapamycin or mTOR pathway. The mTOR pathway regulates cell division and participates in multiple signaling pathways, which are involved in such different diseases as cancer, arthritis, insulin resistance, and osteoporosis. By inhibiting the mTOR pathway through caloric restriction, more energy can be used for self-repair processes, thus extending an animal's life. One of these self-repair processes is autophagy, in which dysfunctional components of a cell are broken down, removed, and even recycled.

The mTOR pathway was discovered when researchers made an expedition to Easter Island and collected soil samples among the large stones. What they discovered was a bacterium that produces an antifungal chemical. Further research later identified a substance called rapamycin, which is now an important immune suppressant drug used in cancer treatment and organ transplants. The name rapamycin was given to acknowledge its discovery on Easter Island, whose Polynesian name is Rapa Nui.

One anti-aging supplement suggested by Sinclair is metformin, an effective type 2 diabetic drug which also inhibits the mTOR pathway. Metformin also affects the AMP-activated protein kinase or AMPK pathway. The AMPK pathway coordinates cell growth, autophagy, and metabolism. In addition, AMPK regulates whole body energy metabolism by telling cells when to store and when to use existing energy reserves. When this pathway becomes activated, it also increases the level of NAD and enlivens SIRT1 enzymes. Calorie restriction and vigorous exercise activate the AMPK pathway, causing fat stores to be used, and producing other beneficial effects that increase the lifespan of animals.

Intermittent Fasting

Many people have tried intermittent fasting or other variations of caloric restriction where, instead of limiting the number of calories, the overall time period for eating is limited to about 8 hours. Typically, intermittent fasting participants stop eating during a 14- to 16-hour period, often skipping either dinner or breakfast. Research on intermittent fasting has provided evidence of improvements in physiological factors such as blood glucose levels and lipid profile, suggesting its value for health. It has also been shown to activate sirtuin pathways.

A major problem among the elderly is not eating enough. Sometimes their appetites diminish and they just choose to eat less. Other times they pick the wrong foods and do not get enough critical vitamins, minerals, essential amino acids, and essential fatty acids. An even more frequent problem is that their guts are inflamed, and they are unable to absorb important nutrients. Reducing caloric intake or doing intermittent fasting may be completely inappropriate for these undernourished individuals who may require the attention of a qualified physician or other health expert to improve their nutritional intake.

Ayurveda

The idea of eating less and fasting is present in every natural health system tradition, including Ayurveda. Ayurveda also includes recommendations of very specific times when to eat. We will consider more about Ayurvedic dietary advice in Biohack #6.

From Biohack to Habit

Let's say you want to try intermittent fasting. How can you make this biohack a habit? To complete your Biohack Map and Plan follow the steps below using the graphic.

Step 1: Enter your main intention or desire for your biohack in the center.

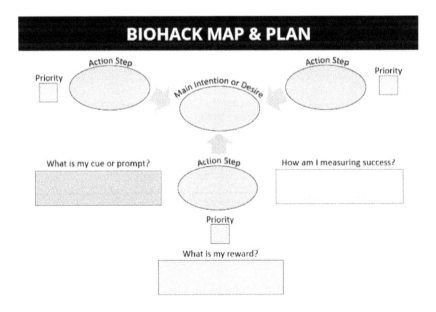

Step 2: Around the central idea for the biohack enter some action steps that you think will help accomplish your change.

Step 3: Prioritize your list and choose the main action step that you want to use.

Step 4: Enter a cue or prompt that will help you remember to do your new action step.

Step 5: Determine how you will measure your success with the new biohack and create a reward.

Step 6: Use feedback from self coaching, personal coaching, group coaching, and environmental coaching to keep improving your ability to adopt new habits.

BIOHACK #5

LONGEVITY SUPPLEMENTS

We have already mentioned a few anti-aging or longevity supplements, but there are many more now available. We will start with a list of well-known modern supplements that include vitamins and minerals most experts agree are important. Then, we will consider modern experimental supplements for longevity, which are more controversial. Finally, we will list ancient Ayurveda longevity supplements that are time-tested and scientifically verified. We give a grade (A to C-) for the quality of research done through animal studies and for human studies. We will also include whether the price of the supplements is either reasonable or high.

Commonly Used Modern Longevity Supplements

#1 Vitamin B12

This is the most obvious longevity supplement because our body does not produce it and yet it is essential for our health. Vegans and other vegetarians often don't get enough B12, since it is mainly found in animal products. A lack of this vitamin can lead to serious health consequences, such as pernicious anemia.

Scientific Evidence in Animals: A

Scientific Evidence in Humans: A

Cost: Reasonable, but sometimes high

2 Vitamin D

If you don't go out in the sun, you may have a problem with a lack of Vitamin D, which is essential for the absorption of calcium and phosphorus, and for maintaining healthy bones and teeth. It also helps with the functioning of the immune system, and it is thought to play a beneficial role in certain physical and mental disorders. The form known as vitamin D3 is usually recommended, but D2 is also effective. The big question is the dose. When taking supplements, it is possible to take too much and elevate your calcium levels so high that you create unwanted side effects. Check with your health expert and be tested regularly.

Scientific Evidence in Animals: A

Scientific Evidence in Humans: A

Cost: Reasonable, but sometimes high.

3 Vitamin C

Vitamin C is a well-known antioxidant and has many crucial functions for healthy aging. Studies confirm, for example, that it reduces the severity and duration of a cold. Another study of elderly adults showed that those with higher blood levels of Vitamin C performed better on mental tasks involving attention and memory.

Scientific Evidence in Animals: A

Scientific Evidence in Humans: A

Cost: Reasonable, but occasionally high

#4 Zinc

Zinc is an essential trace mineral, that acts as a cofactor for over 300 different enzymes and plays a critical role in many important functions in the body. Zinc deficiency has been associated with both disease and aging.

Scientific Evidence in Animals: A

Scientific Evidence in Humans: A

Cost: Reasonable

5 Multivitamin and Mineral Supplements

A good supplement which includes the recommended daily dose of a range of vitamins and minerals is helpful to ensure better health and aging.

Scientific Evidence in Animals: A

Scientific Evidence in Humans: A

Cost: Reasonable, but occasionally high

6 Antioxidants

Many vitamins, such as Vitamin E, Vitamin A, beta carotene, and Vitamin C, are antioxidants. Antioxidants may help repair tissue damage, but the latest research shows that they do not extend life.

Scientific Evidence in Animals: A

Scientific Evidence in Humans: C

Cost: Reasonable

7 Fiber

We don't normally think of fiber as a supplement, so including it here may be going too far. Fiber, however, is definitely good for you and your microbiome and is often lacking in many people's diets. Vegetables, whole grains, fruits, nuts, and seeds are the best natural sources of fiber.

Scientific Evidence in Animals: A

Scientific Evidence in Humans: A

Cost: Reasonable

#8 Probiotic

Probiotics are the subject of the most active areas of research and it is clear that for many people probiotics have helped in a number of different digestive disorders. They are a part of many health traditions, and currently a large number of clinical trials are studying their effects on different disorders. Do probiotics extend our lifespan? We still don't know.

Scientific Evidence in Animals: A

Scientific Evidence in Humans: B

Cost: Reasonable, but sometimes high

Modern Experimental Longevity Supplements

1 Metformin

Metformin is a common and often effective medication for type 2 diabetes that has recently gotten the interest of scientists studying aging. It may have anti-aging properties but the scientific evidence that it extends lifespan in humans is not conclusive. It is also known to have side effects which can include abdominal pain, bloating, diarrhea, nausea, and vomiting.

Scientific Evidence in Animals: A

Scientific Evidence in Humans: B+

Cost: Reasonable

2 EGCG and L-theanine

EGCG (epigallocatechin gallate) and L-theanine are natural antioxidants that are present in green tea. Research has shown anti-cancer, anti-obesity, anti-diabetes, and anti-inflammatory, as well as neuroprotective, effects, and benefits such as improving cardiovascular health and protecting against diabetes. The most obvious way to take these supplements is by drinking green tea.

Scientific Evidence in Animals: A

Scientific Evidence in Humans: B+

Cost: Reasonable

3 Omega-3s

Omega-3 fatty acids have been studied extensively with

conflicting results. More recent reviews have attributed these discrepancies to several factors, including dosage. Omega-3s are currently believed to offer anti-aging benefits such as reducing chronic inflammation, and a lowered risk for heart attack and death from coronary heart disease.

Scientific Evidence in Animals: A

Scientific Evidence in Humans: B

Cost: Reasonable

4 Curcumin

Curcumin (diferuloylmethane) is both modern and ancient. It is the active ingredient in the ayurvedic herb turmeric. Research on curcumin is more extensive than on many other natural products. Studies on curcumin have also shown it affects the expression of SIRT1 protein, suggesting a positive role in the treatment of diabetes, heart disease, and aging. While numerous benefits in animals have been found in thousands of published papers, human studies are limited by the bioavailability of this active ingredient. A 2017 study points out that no double-blind, placebo-controlled clinical trials of curcumin have ever shown conclusive results. It further states that when curcumin is isolated, it is unstable, reactive, and difficult to assimilate in humans. Is isolating the active ingredient the best approach when there could be other beneficial substances in turmeric that interact synergistically to enhance its absorption and overall effects?

Scientific Evidence in Animals: A

Scientific Evidence in Humans: C-

Cost: Reasonable

5 Resveratrol

Resveratrol, derived from grape skins, stimulates the SIRT1 protein. Studies have shown that the combination of resveratrol and caloric restriction can markedly extend the lifespan of animals. But resveratrol is not assimilated very well in humans, and, like many other anti-aging substances, it isn't always effective.

Scientific Evidence in Animals: A

Scientific Evidence in Humans: C-

Cost: Reasonable

6 Quercetin

Quercetin has been seen to increase SIRT1 activity by five times, and acts as a senolytic, a compound that can eliminate old or senescent cells whose presence adversely affect other cells and accelerate the aging process. Most of the results have been found in animals and not humans.

Scientific Evidence in Animals: A

Scientific Evidence in Humans: C-

Cost: Reasonable

7 Rapamycin

Rapamycin is an immune suppressant that has been found to increase the lifespan of animals but may be too potent for humans.

Scientific Evidence in Animals: A

Scientific Evidence in Humans: C-

Cost: High

8 Fisetin

Fisetin is an antioxidant bioactive flavonoid compound found in fruits and vegetables that acts as a senolytic, killing senescent cells. Animal studies suggest that it may reduce the number of senescent cells in tissues, extend lifespan, and improve cognitive and behavioral performance.

Scientific Evidence in Animals: A

Scientific Evidence in Humans: C

Cost: Reasonable

9 NAD

The longevity supplement NAD is known to energize the sirtuin pathway and boost the activity of all 7 sirtuin proteins (SIRT1 through SIRT7). Precursor compounds such as nicotinamide riboside (NR) and nicotinamide mononucleotide (NMN) may help create NAD in the body that could be beneficial to healthy aging. Clinical trials have shown its safety and the effectiveness of the precursor vitamin, nicotinamide riboside (NR), in stimulating NAD metabolism in healthy middle-aged and older adults. Further human studies are needed.

Scientific Evidence in Animals: A

Scientific Evidence in Humans: C-

Cost: High

10 CoQ10

CoQ10 is an antioxidant produced naturally by your body. CoQ10 declines with age. It is involved in the growth and maintenance of cells and has been suggested to help with treating congestive heart failure and a variety of other conditions. Supplements are often made with ubiquinone, an already-oxidized form of CoQ10 that is difficult for your body to absorb. Other formulations are attempting to improve bioavailability.

Scientific Evidence in Animals: A

Scientific Evidence in Humans: C-

Cost: Reasonable

Ancient Ayurveda Longevity Supplements

#1 Amrit Kalash

There is a section of knowledge in Ayurveda known as rasayanas, which are biohacks for longevity. One of the most important of these anti-aging compounds is Maharishi Amrit Kalash, which has been extensively studied. Its chemical analysis shows that it contains plant phytochemicals with strong antioxidant properties that include polyphenols, bioflavonoids, Vitamins C and E, beta carotene, catechin, tannic acid, and resveratrol. Maharishi Amrit Kalash is recommended to be taken as two separate compounds, "Nectar", and "Ambrosia." It is composed of 23 herbs.

There has been extensive scientific research on Maharishi

Amrit Kalash at institutions such as the US National Institutes of Health, the National Cancer Institute, the Niwa Institute of Immunology in Japan, Ohio State University College of Medicine, Loyola University Medical School, University of Kansas Medical Center, South Dakota State University, University of Colorado, Indiana University, SRI International, and the University of California at Irvine.

The studies have shown the rasayana Maharishi Amrit Kalash to have important potential benefits:

- inhibiting tumor growth

- reducing free radicals

- positively influencing known cardiovascular risk factors

- inhibiting degenerative processes, including abnormal platelet aggregation (clotting leading to cardiovascular disease) and the aging process

- enhancing immune response

This preparation and other rasayanas have been time-tested over many hundreds of years. According to Ayurveda, this herbal preparation helps to reset the proper sequential unfoldment of the inner intelligence of the body, and automatically corrects imbalances that may lead to disease.

Scientific Evidence in Animals: A

Scientific Evidence in Humans: B

Cost: Reasonable to High

#2 Triphala

Triphala is classified as a tridoshic rasayana. It is an important Ayurvedic preparation which contains the following three medicinal fruits:

amalaki or amla (*Emblica officinalis,* or Indian gooseberry)

bibhitaki (*Terminalia bellirica*)

haritaki (*Terminalia chebula*)

Animal research on Triphala has found many potential beneficial properties which include being anti-inflammatory, acting as an appetite stimulant, helping gastric hyperacidity, preventing dental caries, and having anticancer and chemopreventive effects. It has been studied extensively for its use in gastrointestinal health and is commonly used to reduced constipation and flatulence while improving the consistency of bowel movements. It also has unique properties of reducing stress and improving cardiovascular health.

Scientific Evidence in Animals: A

Scientific Evidence in Humans: B+

Cost: Reasonable

#3 Ashwagandha

One of the primary uses of Ashwagandha (Withania somnifera) is in reducing stress and improving mental alertness in older individuals. Studies have shown reduced anxiety, depression, and improvements in insomnia and overall well-being.

Scientific Evidence in Animals: A

Scientific Evidence in Humans: B

Cost: Reasonable

#4 Brahmi

An important herb in Ayurveda is Brahmi (*Bacopa monieri*). Animal studies have shown clear anti-inflammatory properties. Other studies have shown improvements in cognitive function such as learning, attention, and memory as well as its role in improving the body's ability to deal with stress.

Scientific Evidence in Animals: A

Scientific Evidence in Humans: B

Cost: Reasonable

FDA Approval

Although supplements show promising results in animals, very few well-controlled clinical studies have proven their effectiveness in humans. One obstacle to good human studies is the high cost. The final step for the approval of any supplement into our modern health system involves the Food and Drug Administration (FDA). Before any substance is advertised or prescribed as a drug that can be used to treat or cure a particular disease, it must go through a rigorous series of tests and clinical trials. Conclusive phase III clinical trials can cost billions of dollars and drug companies invest in these trials based on their expectation of receiving a large return once the drug is approved. If the substance is a natural product that is widely available at very low cost, there is no incentive for a drug company to make such an investment. The very system we have created to protect us from the adverse side effects of modern drugs makes the approval of natural products extremely difficult.

From Biohack to Habit

Let's say you want to try a longevity supplement. How can you make this biohack a habit? To complete your Biohack Map and Plan follow the steps below using the graphic.

Step 1: Enter your main intention or desire for your biohack in the center.

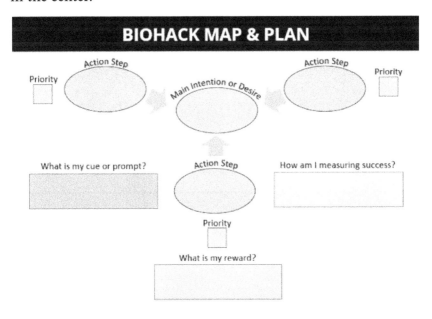

Step 2: Around the central idea for the biohack enter some action steps that you think will help accomplish your change.

Step 3: Prioritize your list and choose the main action step that you want to use.

Step 4: Enter a cue or prompt that will help you remember to do your new action step.

Step 5: Determine how you will measure your success with the new biohack and create a reward.

Step 6: Use feedback from self coaching, personal coaching, group coaching, and environmental coaching to keep improving your ability to adopt new habits.

BIOHACK #6

DIET

How important is diet for longevity? In traditional medicine it is everything. In modern medicine it has only recently become important. In the past the biggest concern with diet was for those who are obese since obesity is a risk factor for heart disease and diabetes. With the discovery of the microbiome, however, diet has gained more significance because our diet alters our gut microbiome, and the gut microbiome has been implicated in numerous disorders.

Dietary Recommendations

Should we follow a Mediterranean, Paleo, vegan, or Ketogenic diet? The *US News and World Report* considers the DASH and Mediterranean diets as the healthiest. DASH stands for Dietary Approach to Stop Hypertension, and includes lots of fruits, vegetables, whole grains, lean proteins, and low-fat dairy. It also recommends reducing salt, saturated fats, and high-sugar or artificially sweetened drinks. The Mediterranean diet is similar, with a few variations. The main feature of the Mediterranean diet is that it includes olive oil, legumes, unrefined cereals, fruits, and vegetables, with a moderate consumption of fish, dairy products (mostly cheese and yogurt), wine, and fewer meat products.

The most common and consistent recommendation among alternative health experts is to eat locally grown, organic and non-GMO foods. They also warn against the perils of gluten, dairy, and sugar, and often recommend a diet like the Keto diet. The ketogenic diet is a very low-carb, high-fat diet that generally eliminates gluten, dairy, and sugar, although there are variations and exceptions. The idea is to put the body into a state of ketosis in which you burn fat for fuel for most of the body. The brain is unable to use fat but if you turn fats in the liver into ketones they can then be used by the brain for energy. While not everyone is up to the Keto or other more radical diets, there are many people trying gluten-free, sugar-free, and dairy-free diets. The Gallup Poll estimates that one in five Americans is experimenting with gluten-free products while the number of people who avoid wheat and other grains containing gluten continually rises.

One of the big problems with dairy is lactose intolerance. Lactose is composed of two simple sugars, glucose and galactose. When you were a baby, you produced an enzyme called lactase, which breaks the lactose into glucose and galactose—a necessary step to allow these sugars to be absorbed into the cells of your small intestine. Over time, however, and depending on your genetic make-up, many people stop making the enzyme lactase. Approximately 75% of all African Americans, Native Americans, and Jewish Americans are lactose intolerant, along with 50% of Mexican Americans and 90% of Asian Americans. About 90% of Americans of Northern European descent are able to produce the enzyme lactase even as adults, and are therefore able to absorb the milk sugar into their bloodstream.

If lactose isn't digested in the small intestine, it goes to the large intestine, where it is fermented by the gut bacteria. The result is excess gas, causing abdominal pain, bloating, and other intestinal problems. Each individual is different and there may be periods in your life during which you may be more or less sensitive to dairy. Medical tests and experts can help to evaluate whether you are lactose intolerant or allergic to milk proteins.

Sugar is a highly controversial topic among alternative health experts. Some recommend that you eliminate it completely from your diet. The American Heart Association conducted a highly comprehensive study on sugar, which led to the conclusion that excess sugar increases the risk of developing obesity, cardiovascular disease, hypertension, and obesity-related cancers. They now recommend that children consume less sugar as part of a healthier diet. Shamefully, the food industry still helps fund many important health associations, such as the American Heart Association and the American Diabetic Association. An article in The *New York Times* revealed that Coca-Cola, the world's largest producer of sugary beverages, has provided millions of dollars in funding for researchers to play down the link between sugary drinks and obesity.

Fructose is a simple sugar present in fruits, Now it is

commercially produced as high-fructose corn syrup and added to drinks and all kinds of food. It turns out that about 40% of the population has trouble digesting and absorbing fructose, a condition called fructose malabsorption. (This is not to be confused with hereditary fructose intolerance, which is a far more serious condition caused by a deficiency of certain enzymes in the liver.) A piece of apple pie might not bother us, but when we have it with a soda containing high-fructose corn syrup, it is too much for the small intestine to absorb. Instead, it goes down into the colon where it is fermented by the gut bacteria that produce excess gas. This excess gas often results in abdominal pain and bloating, along with either diarrhea or constipation.

Modern Digestive Disorders

One of the clearest signs that diet and digestion are affecting health and longevity is the rise of Irritable Bowel Syndrome (IBS). IBS is the number one digestive disorder in the US, affecting between 25 and 45 million people of all ages, 2 out of 3 of whom are women. If you don't have IBS, you probably know someone who does. This disorder can have multiple and sometimes conflicting symptoms, such as an alternation between diarrhea and constipation. You may also have indigestion, excess gas and bloating, or nausea. IBS can be both uncomfortable and debilitating. It is often accompanied by unpredictable abdominal pain, which can be problematic for your professional and social life. The exact cause of this disorder is unknown, but many factors contribute to it, including diet, stress, and imbalanced gut bacteria. IBS has been treated by probiotics with some success.

Leaky Gut Syndrome

Another major digestive disorder is Leaky Gut Syndrome which for a long time was only recognized and treated by alternative health experts. This condition is recognized by a range of digestive symptoms that include gas, bloating, cramps, nausea, indigestion, heartburn, and food sensitivity. Much of what is now understood about a leaky gut comes from the work of Dr. Alessio Fasano, one of the world's leading experts on celiac disease. Dr. Fasano has shown that gluten in wheat contains a short protein called gliadin, which triggers a series of biochemical events that cause a leaky gut. The cells that line the walls of our small intestine are normally held together by tight junctions (which consist of specialized proteins that bind the cells as a rope might bind two pieces of wood). In a healthy state, a tight junction allows only water and very small particles to go from the gut into your bloodstream and throughout your body. But if you have celiac disease and you eat wheat, the gliadin causes these junctions to momentarily come apart.

In these patients, even a tiny amount of gliadin can trigger a long-term opening in the tight junctions, which creates a "leaky gut." When the gut lining is breached, larger molecules and even bacteria can enter your bloodstream and cause an inflammatory response. If a celiac patient continues to consume foods that contain gluten, the result is chronic inflammation and even a full-blown autoimmune response, during which the immune system becomes so agitated that it begins to attack normal, healthy body tissues. The only real solution for a celiac patient is to stop eating anything containing gluten—wheat, barley, rye, etc.

Ayurveda

In traditional systems of medicine such as Ayurveda, diet and digestion are the most important factors for health and longevity. Food is regarded as medicine. There are three fundamental concepts which are critical to understanding diet and digestion in Ayurveda: *agni*, *ama*, and *dosha*. Each of these plays a huge role in health and longevity.

Agni refers to the fire of digestion. In modern medicine, we might equate agni with the digestive enzymes that break down various types of foods, as well as enzymes controlling metabolism in different cells. The agni in your lower gut correlates with the gut bacteria present in the large intestine.

Ama is food that has not been properly broken down and digested. If your agni is weak, ama accumulates and clogs your system, causing health problems. It is particularly harmful when it leaves the digestive system and enters other parts of the body, accumulating in the tissues. Symptoms of excess ama include fatigue and a feeling of heaviness, congestion, constipation, and mental confusion or "brain fog." Ayurveda considers excess ama to be the root cause of all disease. This is a concept similar to leaky gut, where food that has not been digested properly leaks into the bloodstream and aggravates the immune system, creating health problems.

Doshas

The meaning of dosha is not easily translated into modern language. In Sanskrit the word literally translates as "fault" or "defect." In Ayurveda, the three doshas are referred to as three basic energies which maintain the body. How can it be a fault and a basic energy? The idea is that when the doshas accumulate abnormally, they cause disease. When they are in balance, they act as forces or energies which underly all bodily functions. In the quiz in Chapter 1, we talked about the three doshas—Vata, Pitta, and Kapha—as V, P, and K Energy States.

Vata refers to all the functions and systems of the body that control movement, including the nervous system. Pitta refers to the bodily functions concerned with metabolism, such as the digestive system. Kapha refers to those functions involved with structure and lubrication, such as the bones and joints.

At birth each of us has our own individual nature or Prakriti, which is a combination of the three doshas. This is similar to the genes we are born with. At any given time in our life an ayurvedic physician, or Vaidya, can assess your Vikriti, which refers to the current state of balance of all three doshas. In terms of modern science, we can think of this as the immediate state of gene expression during which certain genes are turned on and off. We know from epigenetics that everything in our environment, including diet, can turn genes on and off. By knowing our Prakriti and Vikriti, an ayurvedic Vaidya can personalize recommendations for our diet, lifestyle, and herbs to prevent disease, maintain health, and extend our life.

People with a primarily Vata constitution or V Energy State, have a variable digestion. When the Vata digestion is out of balance, they often become constipated, and may produce gas. Vata individuals tend to have a sensitive gut and are more susceptible to minor disruptions. Stress easily affects their mental state, causing worry, anxiety, and fear.

Pittas, P Energy State people, have a strong digestion. If they are imbalanced or stressed, however, they can have a hyper-acidic stomach. In terms of emotional balance, the seemingly simple act of not eating on time can make them irritable and even angry

Kaphas, K Energy State individuals, are described in Ayurveda as having a slower digestion and metabolism. When imbalanced, they can overeat and easily gain weight. An imbalance in Kapha can also lead to a lethargic and depressed state of mind.

Ayurvedic General Principles

The following are some general principles of digestion for

all dosha combinations on how to eat. Ayurveda recommendations include:

- Eat your main meal at noon when your digestive power is strongest.

- Always sit when you eat.

- Eat in a settled environment and avoid stimulation, such as the TV or telephone, or heated emotional conversations at the table.

- Eat when you are hungry.

- Don't overeat—fill up to approximately ¾ capacity.

- Before, during, and after a meal, avoid cold water and especially ice because cold liquids reduce the fire of digestion.

- Sip small amounts of room temperature or warm water with your meal instead.

- Remain seated for about five minutes after you have finished eating, this will help your digestion.

- Take enough time to digest one meal before starting the next and avoid snacking between meals.

- Different foods and spices are prescribed to balance each Energy State.

- It's ideal to eat organic food rather than taking in

more toxins in the form of synthetic pesticides and fertilizers.

- It is good to avoid GMO (genetically modified) foods but don't strain, do the best you can to eat pure, delicious food.

- The freshness of food is of great importance in Ayurveda.

- Since Ayurveda recommends regular detoxing and improving digestion, it is good to periodically go on a cleansing diet.

- Ayurveda recommends natural probiotics that are helpful for the health of the gut microbiome.

These guidelines and the recommendations below are from the book *The Rest and Repair Diet* which combines principles from Ayurveda with modern ideas about health. The Rest and Repair diet is designed to detox your gut, allow it to repair itself, and improve digestion and health.

Vata Diet

- Favor foods that have a sweet, sour, or salty taste.

- Avoid foods that have a pungent, bitter, or astringent taste.

- Eat on a regular schedule.

- Favor warm, unctuous foods because they're easier to digest and assimilate.

- Avoid light, dry, and cold foods.

- Use oils frequently and generously. Butter, especially clarified butter or ghee, and olive oil are very good.

- Sip hot water throughout the day to promote natural detoxing and improve digestion.

- An ideal breakfast is cooked cereal with roasted nuts and a little fruit. If you're gluten intolerant, pick appropriate non-gluten grains.

- Roasted nuts and seeds are good, especially almonds. It's best not to eat raw nuts, but we can only do what we can do. Roasting nuts helps with digestion and assimilation. Ayurveda recommends first soaking them overnight and then roasting.

- All fresh organic dairy products are highly recommended.

- A modest amount of any natural sweetener helps to calm Vata.

- Hot cooked food is better for a Vata than cold or uncooked food. Small leafy salads, however, are OK.

- Favor rice and, if you can, wheat, and oats (cooked, not dry).

- Eating fresh corn in season is fine! Otherwise, not so much.

- Reduce your intake of millet, barley, buckwheat, and rye.

- A Vata is vulnerable to excess gas, so reduce the intake of all bean products accordingly. (Tofu is hard to digest. But if you love it, then take small amounts, and only if it's very fresh.)

- Fruits should be very ripe, sweet, and juicy!

- For non-vegetarians, favor fresh organic chicken, turkey, fish, and eggs.

- Avoid stimulants like coffee, tea, and other caffeine-laden beverages. Try to cool it on the alcohol.

- If you've been using skim milk to reduce your fat intake, ayurvedic doctors recommend that you buy organic whole milk and dilute it with purified water. This will reduce your fat intake but will also ensure that you benefit from the important synergistic value of all the nutrients in the milk.

- If you're not sleeping well, cook a cup of whole milk for several minutes (ideally, bring it to a boil four times). While the milk is cooking, add cardamom, cinnamon, nutmeg, and coconut sugar, to taste. Drink while it's still nicely warm, but not too hot. If you find that the milk clogs you up overnight, then add a little powdered ginger to the mix. (Too much ginger can be over-stimulating and keep you up or give you a stomachache.)

- **Best veggies**: asparagus, beets, cucumbers, green beans, okra, radishes, sweet potatoes, turnips, carrots, and artichokes. Other vegetables may be eaten in moderation if cooked in ghee (clarified butter) or extra-virgin olive oil. Avoid or reduce cabbage, cauliflower, Brussels sprouts, or bean sprouts. No raw vegetables except for small leafy salads.

- **Best fruits**: apricots, plums, berries, melons, papayas, peaches, cherries, nectarines, and bananas. Also good are dates, figs, pineapples, and mangoes. If you have digestive problems, fruits are best eaten lightly stewed or sautéed. Avocados (technically a fruit) are very good for Vatas.

- **Best spices**: basil, cardamom, cilantro, cinnamon, clove, cumin, fennel, fenugreek, ginger, licorice root, marjoram, nutmeg, oregano, sage, tarragon, and thyme. Allspice, anise, asafoetida, bay leaf, caraway, juniper berries, mace, and mustard can be used with discretion. Use black pepper sparingly. Minimize or eliminate all bitter and astringent spices.

Pitta Diet

- Sweet, bitter, astringent, cold, heavy, and dry foods are

best for a Pitta.

- Avoid pungent, sour, salty, hot, oily, and light foods, which will imbalance and inflame Pitta.

- All natural sweeteners may be taken in moderation, except for molasses and honey, which are both heating to the physiology.

- Favor foods that are cooling in nature, avoiding excessive stimulants like caffeine and very spicy foods.

- Favor ghee (clarified butter), butter (non-salted), milk, and ice cream.

- Since sour tastes irritate a Pitta, sour or fermented products like yogurt, sour cream, and cheese should be taken sparingly, if at all.

- Organic grains like wheat, rice, barley, and oats are good. Reduce your consumption of corn, rye, millet, and brown rice.

- Most nuts are not good for a Pitta. Pumpkin seeds and sunflower seeds are alright.

- Favor organic coconut, olive, and sunflower oils.

- Avoid almond, corn, safflower, and sesame oils.

- Favor mung beans and chickpeas.

- Tofu and other soy products should be fresh. (In Japan, it's not uncommon for people to refuse tofu products that are more than a day old.)

- For non-vegetarians, organic free-range chicken and turkey are preferable to red meat and seafood.

- **Best veggies**: asparagus, potatoes, sweet potatoes, leafy greens, broccoli, cauliflower, celery, okra, lettuce, green beans, peas, and zucchini. Also good are Brussels sprouts, cabbage, cucumbers, mushrooms, sprouts, and sweet peppers. Avoid or reduce tomatoes, hot peppers, onions, garlic, and hot radishes.

- **Best fruits**: apples, grapes, melons, cherries, coconuts, avocados, mangoes, pineapples, figs, oranges, and plums are recommended. Also good are prunes, and raisins. Reduce or eliminate sour fruits such as grapefruit, cranberries, lemons, and persimmons.

- **Best spices**: coriander, cilantro, cardamom, and saffron. Turmeric, dill, fennel, and mint are also fine. Spices such as ginger, black pepper, fenugreek, clove, salt, and mustard seed may be used sparingly. Completely *avoid* pungent hot spices such as chili peppers and cayenne.

Kapha Diet

- Pungent, bitter, and astringent, as well as light, hot, and dry foods, are best.

- Sweet, sour, salty, heavy, oily, and cold foods have the

opposite, imbalancing effect.

- Enjoy smaller meals that are well-spiced and focus on light foods like quinoa, vegetables, and fruit.

- Favor milk with reduced fat and again note: For you to benefit from the synergistic value of everything in the milk, it is far better to water down whole milk than to use skim milk.

- In general, it's good to reduce dairy intake

- Honey is the only sweetener that helps a Kapha. Avoid all others.

- According to Ayurveda, honey should not be heated.

- Favor barley, corn, millet, buckwheat, and rye.

- Reduce your intake of oats, rice, and wheat.

- Beans of all kinds are good for a Kapha, except kidney beans and soybeans. Soy is quite difficult to digest, and the older it is, the harder it is to digest.

- Except for pumpkin seeds and sunflower seeds, reduce or eliminate the intake of nuts and seeds.

- Use small amounts of extra virgin olive oil, ghee, almond oil, sunflower oil, or safflower oil. Steam or roast, if possible.

- Non-vegetarians should favor fresh organic free-range chicken and turkey.

- **Best veggies**: asparagus, beets, broccoli, Brussels sprouts, cabbage, carrots, cauliflower, celery, eggplant, leafy greens, lettuce, mushrooms, okra, onions, peas, peppers, potatoes, spinach, sprouts
  Use small amounts of ghee or extra-virgin olive oil. Reduce/Avoid: sweet potatoes, tomatoes, cucumbers, zucchini

- **Best fruits**: pomegranates, apples, apricots, cranberries, pears. Reduce/Avoid: avocados, bananas, oranges, peaches, coconuts, melons, dates, figs, grapefruits, grapes, mangoes, papayas, plums, pineapples

- **Best spices**: ginger, horseradish, mustard, cardamom, garlic, cloves, turmeric, cayenne and peppers of all kinds. Ginger is great for improving digestion! Reduce or avoid salt.

From Biohack to Habit

Let's say you want to improve your diet. How can you make this biohack a habit? To complete your Biohack Map and Plan follow the steps below using the graphic.

Step 1: Enter your main intention or desire for your biohack in the center.

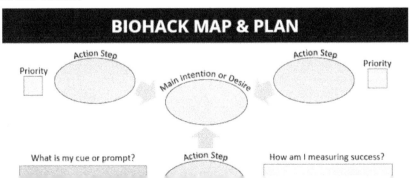

Step 2: Around the central idea for the biohack enter some action steps that you think will help accomplish your change.

Step 3: Prioritize your list and choose the main action step that you want to use.

Step 4: Enter a cue or prompt that will help you remember to do your new action step.

Step 5: Determine how you will measure your success with the new biohack and create a reward.

Step 6: Use feedback from self coaching, personal coaching, group coaching, and environmental coaching to keep improving your ability to adopt new habits.

BIOHACK #7

GUT MICROBIOME

The microbiome is the totality of all the microorganisms (bacteria, fungi, viruses, etc.) that live *in* and *on* you. Our focus here is on the 30 trillion microbes in the lower gut. People used to be afraid of bacteria, but it turns out that most of the bacteria in our gut are friendly. What's even more remarkable is that recent research suggests that the state of our health and longevity depend on the state of these microorganisms. This supports the ancient notion expressed by Hippocrates, the father of western medicine, that "All disease begins in the gut."

Our diet has a significant impact on the composition of the gut bacteria. Switching from a plant-based diet to a meat-based diet or vice versa can quickly change it. Some bacteria prefer certain food while others prefer entirely different types of food. Whichever bacteria get fed the most increase in number and change the ecology of our gut microbiome.

Many of these gut bacteria don't use oxygen, which, for years, made it hard for researchers to study them. With the introduction of gene-sequencing techniques, scientists had a new and relatively inexpensive tool to identify and study them. As a result, the microbiome is an active area of medical research and the subject of hundreds of clinical trials.

Functions of Gut Bacteria

Our gut bacteria help us to digest different types of food. Most nutrients are digested and absorbed in the small intestine, but some foods cannot be digested by the enzymes present there. Fruits and vegetables, for example, contain fiber that passes right through the small intestine and goes into the large intestine, where friendly bacteria digest and ferment the fiber. Some of the important products of this fermentation are short-chain fatty acids (SCFAs) like acetic acid, propionic acid, and butyric acid—a primary source of nutrients and energy for cells lining the colon. SCFAs have many other functions, including helping our body absorb essential minerals like calcium, magnesium, and iron.

Second, our gut bacteria make B vitamins, including thiamine or B1, riboflavin or B2, nicotinic acid (a form of niacin) or B3, pantothenic acid or B5, pyridoxine or B6, biotin or B7, folate (folic acid) or B9, and cobalamin or B12, as well as a certain type of Vitamin K, which is necessary to make special blood clotting factors. Vitamin B12 is an interesting example. It's involved in the metabolism of every cell in our body, and it is especially important to the functioning of our nervous system and the formation of red blood cells. Vitamin B12 is synthesized only by certain bacteria and archaea (microorganisms which are a little more advanced than bacteria), not by plants. Scientists have suggested that the gut bacteria alone are not capable of fulfilling our B12 needs and that other sources of this vitamin are required. The production of B12 in the gut, therefore, is probably more important for the health of the cells in the colon rather than for the rest of our body.

The third important function of gut bacteria is to help protect us from the invasion of harmful microorganisms. It turns out that 70-80% of our total immune system is located in the lining of the gut. Friendly bacteria occupy critical locations along the gut lining so that bad bacteria are prevented from crossing the gut barrier. The friendly or "good" guys also protect us by secreting antimicrobial chemicals to attack and destroy bad bacteria.

The fourth function is that they play a key role in the development of our gut lining. Without these friendly bacteria, certain gut immune and nerve cells do not mature properly, which jeopardizes the health of the entire gut lining.

The fifth function of gut bacteria is that they communicate with many parts of the body. The bacteria are part of the gut-brain axis, which consists of the nervous system, endocrine system, immune system, enteric (gut) nervous system, and enteric endocrine system. One way they communicate is directly through the vagus nerve, and another is indirectly by producing critical substances that can cross the gut barrier and enter the bloodstream, influencing digestion, appetite, state of mind—turning genes on and off throughout your body.

Sixth, an abnormal composition of gut bacteria, called dysbiosis, seem to be involved in many different types of diseases, such as: inflammatory bowel disease, irritable bowel syndrome, colon cancer, allergies, asthma, autoimmune diseases, Parkinson's disease, autism, Alzheimer's, multiple sclerosis, depression, anxiety, type 1 and 2 diabetes, stroke, high blood pressure, high cholesterol, and heart disease. The list grows longer every day.

Finally, the microbiome is important for aging. The microbiome theory of aging attributes the deleterious effects of aging to a disruption of the gut microbiome and a reduction of the diversity of microorganisms. A balanced diet creates a balanced and diverse microbiome.

Factors Influencing Gut Bacteria

The first factor is the way we are born. Does the child come down the birth canal or from a caesarean birth? If a caesarean operation must be performed, the first bacteria to colonize the infant's gut are from the hospital environment; these are frequently not friendly bacteria. Studies show that children from caesarean births have a higher incidence of asthma, allergies, and autoimmune diseases, and a propensity toward obesity in adulthood. In some countries, like China, over 50% of all births are caesarean. In private hospitals in Brazil, the number reaches 80%. Italy has the second highest caesarean birth rate in Europe at 38%, and over 30% of all births in the US are caesarean.

A second factor is antibiotics. Most of us have taken antibiotics at some point in our lives for a bad infection. The problem is that a single dose can wipe out billions of helpful friendly bacteria. Most medical experts now agree that these drugs have been massively overprescribed. One negative side effect of this is that certain bacteria have eventually become resistant to antibiotics, posing a very real health threat, especially in hospitals. We don't know how long it takes for a damaged microbiome to recover from a course of antibiotics. Each person reacts differently; some people can recover completely in a short time while others may lose certain species of bacteria forever.

The third and most important factor that influences our gut bacteria is our diet. One excellent study examined gut bacteria in healthy children between ages one and six, living either in Europe (Italy) or in rural Africa (Burkina Faso), and found striking differences between the two ethnic and cultural groups. Scientists concluded that one of the reasons for these differences was the fiber content in the diet, which was almost twice as high in the children from Burkina Faso as compared to the Italian children. Many studies have extended this research and consistently show that diet is a critical factor in changing our microbial community. Hundreds of clinical studies are underway, seeking to discover whether a specific diet, probiotic, or lifestyle can help to cure specific diseases.

There are other factors such as medication, infection, environmental toxins, whether we smoke or not, how much we exercise, and even seasonal rhythms, all of which can affect our microbiome.

Probiotics and Prebiotics

Probiotics are friendly living bacteria. In 1907, Nobel Prize Laureate Ilya Ilyich Mechnikov promoted probiotics in yogurt as a way to maintain better health and slow the aging process. No one took him seriously then, but today well-controlled clinical trials show that probiotics improve a number of intestinal conditions, including irritable bowel syndrome.

It is also impossible to know what the best probiotic is for each person. We all have a different gut microbiome. Are the bacteria in the probiotic product able to reach the lower intestine where they are most needed, before being digested or destroyed?

Most doctors now recommend that we take probiotics after a course of antibiotics. But probiotics contain relatively few types of bacteria, so it is hard to understand how a few friendly bacteria are able to restore the enormous diversity of the hundreds of types of bacteria normally in our gut. Also, there are some 30 trillion bacteria in our lower digestive tract—and if only a few million probiotic bacteria can make it to this destination, will they be enough to make a change in this very competitive environment? Think of it as sending a small group of well-bred private school children into a gang-ridden inner city and hoping that they will be a positive influence.

What about probiotic labeling? Most companies report the number of bacteria contained in their capsules or pills at the date of manufacture. Unfortunately, different storage conditions will reduce this number so that the actual number of bacteria at the time of consumption is difficult to calculate. The European Commission uses stricter labeling requirements and has placed a ban on putting the word "probiotic" on the packaging of products because they do not feel there is enough scientific evidence to justify any assumed health benefits. The FDA allows the use of the word but has tried to limit the listing of benefits for specific diseases. Despite these restrictions there has been an increase in the use of these products, as well as foods containing probiotics.

Probiotics are one of the hottest areas of research today, even though science doesn't fully understand how or why they work. They are no passing health fad. The National Institutes of Health lists hundreds of human clinical trials presently exploring the effectiveness of probiotics to treat a wide range of diseases including: fibromyalgia, obesity, gastrointestinal function, irritable bowel syndrome, anxiety, depression, asthma, type 2 diabetes mellitus, hyperlipidemia, alcoholic liver disease, hypertension, rheumatoid arthritis, bacterial vaginosis, diverticular disease, respiratory infections in children, atopic dermatitis, fatty liver, lactose intolerance, coronary artery disease, bipolar disorder, antibiotic-associated diarrhea, hypertriglyceridemia, HIV, cancer, and necrotizing enterocolitis in preterm infants with very low body weight. There is even a name for probiotics that can treat mental and emotional disorders—psychobiotics. An entirely new field of medicine is emerging, which focuses exclusively on creating better health through the repair of our gut microbiome.

Prebiotics are types of dietary fiber that feed our friendly bacteria. Some of the most potent prebiotics include asparagus, bananas, barley, oats, cocoa, burdock root, flaxseed, wheat bran, seaweed, Jerusalem artichoke, dandelion greens, garlic, leeks, onions, inulin, gum arabic, and chicory root. Research shows that prebiotics have beneficial effects: improving absorption of calcium and other minerals, boosting the immune system, reducing colorectal cancer risk, improving symptoms in inflammatory bowel disease, and improving digestion and elimination. Research is being done to determine the potential beneficial effects of prebiotics for many diseases.

Ayurveda and the Microbiome

Like many natural systems of medicine, Ayurveda recommends natural probiotics such as yogurt and a special drink called lassi which includes yogurt, water, and spices. In the last biohack, we discussed how, according to Ayurveda, if your agni (digestive fire) is weak, then ama (undigested food and toxins) accumulates and clogs your system, causing health problems. This is also true of digestion in the colon. If the gut microbiome is imbalanced (dysbiosis) digestion won't be complete, and by-products of improper digestion and fermentation can enter the bloodstream and cause problems. Research has shown that individuals with a primary Vata, Pitta, or Kapha nature tend to have a different composition of bacteria in their gut microbiome.

Ayurveda gives excellent advice for improving our microbiome. Eat well and consume fresh fruit and vegetables (lots of fiber) that suit your individual Energy State. Ayurveda also recommends taking periodic opportunities to detox and give your gut a chance to rest, repair itself, and reboot its microbiome, which we talk about in Biohack #10.

From Biohack to Habit

Let's say you want to try something to improve your gut microbiome. How can you make this biohack a habit? To complete your Biohack Map and Plan follow the steps below using the graphic.

Step 1: Enter your main intention or desire for your biohack in the center.

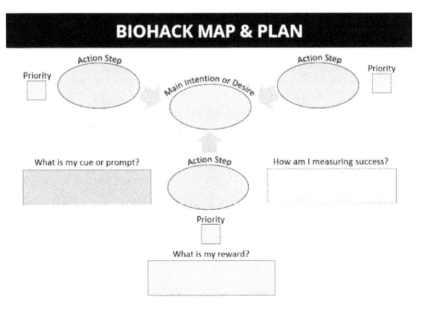

Step 2: Around the central idea for the biohack enter some action steps that you think will help accomplish your change.

Step 3: Prioritize your list and choose the main action step that you want to use.

Step 4: Enter a cue or prompt that will help you remember to do your new action step.

Step 5: Determine how you will measure your success with the new biohack and create a reward.

Step 6: Use feedback from self coaching, personal coaching, group coaching, and environmental coaching to keep improving your ability to adopt new habits.

BIOHACK #8

EXERCISE AND YOGA

Every doctor and health expert agree that exercise is good for your health and longevity. "Walking," said Hippocrates, "is man's best medicine." Research clearly documents that exercise helps in the prevention of chronic diseases including diabetes mellitus, cancer, obesity, hypertension, coronary heart disease, cardiovascular disease, and depression. Physical inactivity is the leading risk factor for cardiovascular disease.

Yet we live in a world where most people don't exercise even when their doctor recommends it. It is estimated that a third of all adults and four-fifths of adolescents, approximately 1.4 billion people, do not meet the recommended criteria for daily and weekly exercise. Many people lie on the couch, not even taking a brief walk, and watch other people exercise. What about retirees who go golfing every day? Sadly, they mostly ride in golf carts and take only a few steps and a few swings. If you are part of this reluctant group, then this is the time to start one simple habit: Take a 15-minute walk each day. If you can do it in the early morning sunlight then you are now practicing habit stacking, which means you have combined two simple habits together— getting sunlight and walking.

What is the best form of exercise? Most experts agree that the best exercise is the one you will do, which differs for each individual. The recommended amount of exercise in order to achieve substantial health benefits is at least 150 to 300 minutes a week (20 to 40 minutes a day) of moderate-intensity physical activity (a brisk walk or doubles tennis), or 75 to 150 minutes a week (10 to 20 minutes a day) of vigorous-intensity aerobic exercise (jogging or a strenuous fitness class) or an equivalent combination of moderate and vigorous exercise. Studies find that people who do team sports may be at an advantage since social interaction often compounds the positive benefits of physical activity.

Can you get too much exercise? Studies have shown that more exercise can be better unless you strain too much and overexercise when you are feeling pain. The sweet spot for longevity lies around 7,000 to 8,000 steps daily (about 30 to 45 minutes of exercise) most days. You can also get this by engaging in sports such as tennis, cycling, swimming, jogging, or badminton, for more than 2.5 hours per week.

Improvements in Mental Health

Regular exercise can have a beneficial effect on depression, anxiety, ADHD, PTSD, and many different mental functions. This may come as a result of the effects of exercise on the brain, as well as the release of endorphins which make you feel good.

Research also shows that exercise promotes gene expression of brain-derived neurotrophic factor (BDNF) in the brain which might account for some of the cognitive and mood improvements.

We now know that skeletal muscles produce small proteins called "myokines," which act on the muscles but can also have endocrine-like effects by traveling through the bloodstream to distant organs such as the brain and liver. Interleukin 6 (IL-6) was one of the first myokines to be discovered, and it has anti-inflammatory and metabolic actions. The muscles also secrete BDNF and other beneficial factors. This new area of research may give us deeper insights into the mechanics of how exercise improves physical and mental health.

Ayurveda and Exercise

Ayurveda prescribes specific types of exercise for different people. If you know your Energy State (included in Biohack #1) then you can tailor all your exercise based on what is best for your Ayurveda Energy State.

V Energy State

V Energy State individuals enjoy exercise that involves moving quickly and/or gracefully; however their physiology is not suited for endurance sports. They are sprinters rather than marathoners and must be very careful to not get overtired. Activities like dancing, walking, cycling, paddleboarding, and yoga are good as well as a gentle-to-moderate, grounding, warming workout.

P Energy State

P Energy State individuals are usually highly competitive and don't hold back. Possessing stamina and strength, they are often drawn to organized sports. They are also goal-oriented and tend to overdo exercise, facing the consequences later. Above all, P people need to avoid becoming overheated. Moderate exercise is recommended including jogging, hiking, winter sports, swimming, Pilates, and strength training. Active water sports like surfing and canoeing are also good for them. If you see people out parasailing, they will almost certainly prove to be P Energy State types.

K Energy State

K Energy State individuals generally have good endurance and strength, and regular active physical exercise helps to keep them from becoming overweight and lethargic (i.e. couch potatoes). Running, jogging, and energetic gym workouts are all beneficial.

Remember, no single Energy State is better than another. We all need to be active.

Yoga Asanas

The word yoga means union, and the ultimate goal of yoga, as expressed in the Vedic tradition, is enlightenment. In the West, we have come to understand yoga as specific yoga postures or asanas, which have become widely practiced. There are many diverse types of yoga and research has shown that yoga postures improve psychological conditions such as anxiety and depression and provide health benefits for those with high blood pressure, various pain syndromes, and immune disorders.

Choose whichever form of yoga best suits your individual nature, age, and needs. We recommend the Maharishi Yoga Asana program because it is especially respectful of your body and supports the experience of transcendence.

From Biohack to Habit

Let's say you want to begin to exercise more. How can you make this biohack a habit? To complete your Biohack Map and Plan follow the steps below using the graphic.

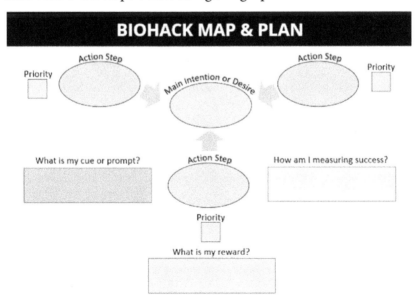

Sept 1: Enter your main intention or desire for your biohack in the center.

Step 2: Around the central idea for the biohack enter some action steps that you think will help accomplish your change.

Step 3: Prioritize your list and choose the main action step that you want to use.

Step 4: Enter a cue or prompt that will help you remember to do your new action step.

Step 5: Determine how you will measure your success with the new biohack and create a reward.

Step 6: Use feedback from self coaching, personal coaching, group coaching, and environmental coaching to keep improving your ability to adopt new habits.

BIOHACK #9

SLEEP

We all know from our experience that if you don't get enough sleep, you'll be tired and unable to focus the next day. But what is enough? There are some who only sleep 5 or 6 hours and have enormous energy the next day and others who need 10 hours and have a tough time getting up in the morning. It is generally agreed that having good sleep habits is a necessary component of health and longevity. What do we mean by good sleep habits? Basically, anything that helps you get the amount of sleep you need. Many studies have shown that when people are deprived of sleep they don't perform well. Studies from shift workers show that those who must sleep during the day have an increased risk of cardio-vascular, metabolic, and neurological disorders.

Detox During Sleep

One of the most interesting new findings about the impor-tance of sleep is that we have a toxin removal system in our brain that works primarily when we are asleep. It is similar to the lymph system in our body, which consists of a set of vessels that run parallel to the blood vessels. One of the most important jobs of the lymph system is the clearance of excess fluid and waste material from the spaces between cells, referred to as the interstitial space. Within the lymph system are lymph nodes, which act like fortresses in which immune cells are constantly checking for any foreign invaders. The materials and fluid in the lymph system are ultimately returned to the general circulation.

But the brain does not have lymph vessels and yet it produces a great deal of metabolic waste. It has its own unique garbage disposal system called the glymphatic system, named by Danish neuroscientist Maiken Nedergaard, who discovered it. A type of glial cell known as astroglia helps allow cerebrospinal fluid (CSF) to move into the interstitial space in the nervous system and clear away waste materials that ultimately are sent to the lymph system. The glymphatic system is largely quiet during waking hours. There are currently many studies investigating the importance of this system in conditions such as Alzheimer's disease in which an excess buildup of waste materials such as beta-amyloid plaques may be the cause of memory loss and other poor cognitive functions.

Melatonin and Other Sleep Aids

One of the most popular sleep supplements is melatonin. Melatonin, as we have learned, is a hormone secreted by the pineal gland and also an antioxidant produced in mitochondria. When it is dark, the pineal gland will naturally produce melatonin, which is why it is called the sleep hormone. When it is light out, as explained in Biohack #3, a pigment in your eyes gets activated and sends signals to the pineal gland to stop producing melatonin. Melatonin also helps regulate specific body functions such as blood temperature, blood glucose, and blood pressure, as well as levels of other hormones.

There are factors which can cause lower melatonin levels at night and inhibit the ability to fall asleep. These include caffeine, alcohol consumption, smoking, shift work, and too much exposure to light at night. Melatonin also decreases with age which may cause sleep problems. Studies do show improvement in sleep onset with melatonin supplements. There can be mild side effects with melatonin, and it doesn't work for everyone particularly over a long period of time. It is generally recommended that you start with a low dose. Other supplements for improving sleep habits include magnesium, tryptophan, L-theanine, and the herbs Valerian and ginkgo biloba. They all have varying results.

Other recommendations for better sleep include taking an early morning walk to reset your circadian rhythms, reducing blue light exposure in the evening, reducing caffeine at night, improving your bedroom environment (less noise, softer lighting, cool temperature, pleasant bedding, etc.), taking a bath before sleeping, and regular exercise (but not right before sleeping).

Ayurveda and Sleep

Ayurveda gives very clear guidelines for sleep habits based on your Energy State. Let's briefly examine these recommendations and then we can outline a more personalized plan for better sleep habits.

V Energy State

V Energy State people frequently have a difficult time going to sleep and are very susceptible to insomnia. They need to understand that they must avoid excessive stimulation before bedtime and take real steps to wind down and relax, such as having a warm bath, listening to peaceful music, and using calming aromatherapy.

P Energy State

A P Energy State person tends to go to sleep quickly. But when the P person goes out of balance, he or she can experience difficulty sleeping and even wake up in the middle of the night.

K Energy State

K Energy State individuals almost never have trouble falling asleep, but they often have a challenging time getting up in the morning.

No matter what your Energy State, Ayurveda recommends going to bed by 10:00 p.m. and waking up early.

From Biohack to Habit

Step 1: Enter your main intention or desire for your biohack in the center.

Step 2: Around the central idea for the biohack enter some action steps that you think will help accomplish your change.

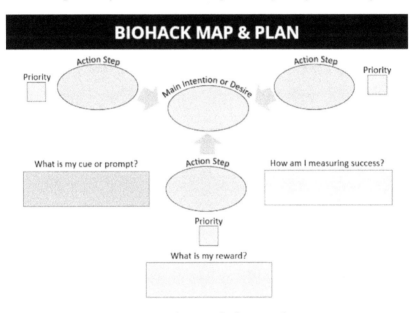

Step 3: Prioritize your list and choose the main action step that you want to use.

Step 4: Enter a cue or prompt that will help you remember to do your new action step.

Step 5: Determine how you will measure your success with the new biohack and create a reward.

Step 6: Use feedback from self coaching, personal coaching, group coaching, and environmental coaching to keep improving your ability to adopt new habits.

BIOHACK #10

DETOX

Detox is a popular topic these days among health aficionados. Do we eat grapefruits for a week or cucumbers? Each one of the detoxes has its own philosophy and very little research has been done on any of them. There are also techniques such as saunas and steam baths that use heat to remove toxins and improve circulation and relaxation. These techniques are beneficial for health and longevity but there are certain precautions to keep in mind such as drinking enough water before using a sauna or steam bath, limiting your time, and if you have any preexisting conditions such as a heart problem, making sure your doctor is comfortable with this form of detox.

Most traditional systems of health, such as Ayurveda, have extensive programs for daily, weekly, and seasonal ways to detox the body. Let's examine some of these.

Ayurveda Daily Detox

One of the simplest is to start the day with a full glass of room temperature water and then use the bathroom for elimination. Throughout the day sip warm or hot water. There are also simple teas that can help you detox. Below is the recipe for a traditional Ayurvedic Digest and Detox Tea. Drink at least three times a day.

- ½ teaspoon organic cumin

- ½ teaspoon fennel

- ½ teaspoon coriander seeds

- 5 cups of hot water

- Boil this mixture for about 5 minutes, strain, and put in a thermos.

One simple detox method to help improve your agni or digestive power is to take a pre-meal digestive aid, which consists of a mixture of fresh ginger juice, lemon juice, and a little salt. If it seems too strong to you, add a little water. To make the digestive aid:

- Grate fresh raw organic ginger

- Put the gratings in a piece of cheese cloth

- Squeeze the juice into a small glass

- Add lemon and salt to taste

Avoid cold drinks (no ice) before, during, and after meals

because cold reduces your digestive fire. You can sip small amounts of warm water with your meal and add a squeeze of lemon for taste.

Finally, at the end of the day use the ayurvedic herbal supplement triphala, which is mentioned in Biohack #5. Take it with warm water, about 30-60 minutes before bed, and this will help with elimination the next day. We have already talked about another approach to detox, intermittent fasting, in Biohack #4.

Weekly and Seasonal Detox

In Ayurveda it is often recommended that a simple detox is having liquids for one day of the week. Remember that for a Vata and a Kapha this can be easy but for a Pitta you really do need to juice some fruits or vegetables and get something of substance in you.

A seasonal Spring detox diet can be of great benefit for all types. Over the winter, according to Ayurveda, Kapha and ama build up in your body. Spring is a period of awakening and renewal, and it is the ideal time to re-balance Kapha and reduce ama to prevent toxins and excess mucus from creating congestion and allergies. It is also the perfect time to reboot and increase your digestive fire or agni, detox your body, repair your gut, and eliminate any excess weight by having a Kapha-reducing diet.

Foods that are primarily Kapha in nature—heavy, greasy, and mucus forming—tend to increase both Kapha and ama. It is important to reduce or eliminate or reduce such Kapha foods as milk products, wheat products, sugar, red meat, nut butters, eggs, chicken, and fish. Kitchari, made from dahl, rice, and specific spices, is one of the healthiest and most beneficial foods to have during a Spring Detox.

In our book *The Rest and Repair Diet* there are several recipes for kitchari and guidelines for a Spring Detox diet. Leafy green vegetables are included because they are good detoxifiers, while heavier root vegetables should be eaten sparingly. It is helpful to note that the bitter, pungent, and astringent tastes of certain foods, spices, and herbs act as a powerful detoxing and cleansing combination. A bitter taste can dry and drain ama, while a pungent taste destroys and digests it.

Panchakarma Detox

In Ayurveda one the most important seasonal detoxes is a treatment called Panchakarma, which means "five actions". The main purpose of panchakarma is to detox, eliminate ama, and remove any obstruction in the body's channels, *srotas*. Panchakarma is done in a specialized treatment center where you are first assessed by an ayurvedic doctor or Vaidya. There are many different approaches such as purgation, massage, elimination, special diets, and herbal preparation. Each is prescribed according to the needs of the individual. Panchakarma is often referred to as "rejuvenation therapy." Studies show that Panchakarma improves mental and physical health as well as vitality, well-being, stamina, appetite, and digestion. One study showed that Panchakarma treatment helped to remove specific environmental toxins such as polychlorinated biphenyls (PCBs) from the body.

Probiotic Enemas and Bastis

There are several elimination therapies in Panchakarma. One is a type of steam bath treatment called swedena. Another is a purgatory treatment called virechana. Perhaps the most effective is a type of enema, called basti. There are two main groups of bastis. One is a nourishing basti and the other an eliminating or purifying basti. The nourishing basti uses oils and other substances to nourish and balance the cells of the colon. The purifying basti is mostly water with some herbs and a little fat. You usually alternate between the two, one day a nourishing basti, the next an eliminating basti.

Bastis can use many different ingredients such as sesame oil and medicated ghee, and a wide variety of herbs. There are many published studies on bastis and their use for various clinical conditions. Bastis often use sesame oil which we know has a positive effect on colon cells and promotes beneficial bacteria.

Dr. David Perlmutter, a qualified neurologist with several best-selling books and a PBS series, talks about using probiotic enemas to help cure certain neurological disorders in his book *Brain Maker*. A probiotic enema provides an almost instantaneous boost to the colon, where most of your gut bacteria live.

Dr. Perlmutter describes Christopher, a teenage boy who had Tourette's syndrome since he was six. Tourette's patients typically have periodic spontaneous and uncontrollable movements, and they tend to repeat certain words or sounds. Over 100,000 children in the U.S. have Tourette's, more than five times as many boys as girls. Although Christopher was able to attend school, by the time he was 13 he was suffering from the social stigma associated with his involuntary movements.

When Dr. Perlmutter interviewed Christopher's mother, facts came to light that pointed to his gut as the source of his disease. First, the boy's Tourette's symptoms worsened after eating specific foods, and secondly, Christopher had received numerous antibiotics when he was young.

Dr. Perlmutter reasoned that Christopher's medical history indicated a massive disruption of his gut bacteria and recommended that the boy take probiotic enemas rather than oral probiotics. The morning after Christopher's first probiotic enema, his mother called to report that her son's body had become noticeably calmer. Under Dr. Perlmutter's supervision, the treatment was continued daily, and the probiotic dosage was increased to 1200 billion units. Christopher's Tourette's symptoms virtually disappeared (Please note: It is important to have your doctor's approval before beginning a probiotic enema program).

Our modern understanding of the gut microbiome helps us understand why bastis were considered by Ayurveda to be so important for the prevention and treatment of chronic diseases. They understood the importance of the digestive system and how to quickly rebalance and help repair it by introducing herbs and oils directly into the colon where the largest number of gut bacteria reside.

From Biohack to Habit

Let's say you want to try a detox program. How can you make this biohack a weekly or seasonal habit? To complete your Biohack Map and Plan follow the steps below using the graphic.

Step 1: Enter your main intention or desire for your biohack in the center.

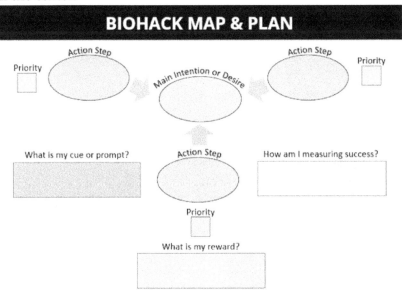

Step 2: Around the central idea for the biohack enter some action steps that you think will help accomplish your change.

Step 3: Prioritize your list and choose the main action step that you want to use.

Step 4: Enter a cue or prompt that will help you remember to do your new action step.

Step 5: Determine how you will measure your success with the new biohack and create a reward.

Step 6: Use feedback from self coaching, personal coaching, group coaching, and environmental coaching to keep improving your ability to adopt new habits.

BIOHACK #11

ROUTINE

Almost every cell in our body has a biological clock which keeps track of the daily circadian rhythm. Modern medicine recognizes the importance of daily rhythms to your health to such an extent that the 2017 Nobel Prize in Physiology or Medicine was awarded for research on the genetic basis of biological rhythms. When we get out of sync with nature all kinds of problems arise in our mental and physical health. We have already explained the significance of early morning sunlight to synchronize our central clock with all the many biological clocks located in different tissues. The modern study of biorhythms is called chronobiology. Research has shown that when our rhythms get out of sync with nature we disturb the sleep-waking patterns, and this can lead to many health issues. Even our immune system activity is influenced by the time of day.

One of the most important timing issues for the body is when you eat. If you eat within 2 hours before you normally go to sleep, it can desynchronize the circadian rhythms of certain cells in the intestine and liver from those in the rest of your body.

One study demonstrated how upsetting biorhythms can have

a negative effects on the microbiome and on the health of the animal. The researchers created jet lag in mice by forcing these normally nocturnal animals to stay awake during the day. When the researchers transferred the gut bacteria from jet-lagged mice into germ-free (no gut bacteria) mice, the recipient mice developed both obesity and glucose intolerance.

Ayurveda

Ayurveda and other traditional systems of medicine have emphasized for centuries the importance of staying in tune with nature. Ayurveda identifies daily, seasonal, and lifetime cycles which all play a role in the prevention and treatment of disease. Ayurvedic science divides up the day into six four-hour sections, each one governed by a different dosha.

The Doshas Throughout the Day

Time	Dominant Dosha
6 am – 10 am	Kapha Dosha
10 am – 2 pm	Pitta Dosha
2 pm – 6 pm	Vata Dosha
6 pm – 10 pm	Kapha Dosha
10 pm – 2 am	Pitta Dosha
2 am – 6 am	Vata Dosha

Daily Routine

Let's look at a typical ayurvedic daily routine and how it accounts for the influence of the doshas.

- Wake up with the sun, or even a little before sunrise before the Kapha time of day truly sets in.

- Upon waking, clean your tongue with a metal tongue scraper to clear any white coating (this is the byproduct of your liver's natural cleansing process which takes place between 10 p.m. and 2 a.m. during the transformational Pitta period).

- After cleaning your tongue, drink a glass of warm water to help flush your system and move your bowels. The water should not be cold. You can leave a covered glass of water by your bedside overnight and drink it first thing in the morning.

- Evacuate your bowels. A healthy system eliminates waste every morning. If you are experiencing constipation, add more fruit (raisins, figs, and prunes).

- Ignite your energy through the practice of yoga, pranayama, and meditation. We recommend the twice-daily practice of the Transcendental Meditation technique.

- Keep your energy going by exercising to remove the heaviness of sleep and to promote lymph circulation to improve immunity—a brisk walk will suffice.

- Eat a breakfast appropriate for your Energy State and state of health.

- Use your morning energy to do creative work and continue during the Pitta morning period.

- Eat your main meal at noon during this Pitta period when your digestion is strongest.

- Have an early dinner according to your mind/body type and state of health during this Vata period.

- Go to bed before 10 p.m. during the Kapha period and before the next Pitta period kicks in.

Seasonal and Life Routine

Now let's consider how the doshas affect seasonal routines. Fall and winter are cold and dry and correspond to the combination of Vata and Kapha dosha. Summer is hot and naturally corresponds to Pitta dosha. Spring is cold and wet and corresponds to Kapha dosha. In Biohack #10 on detox, we considered the Spring Detox diet and Panchakarma treatments as part of a seasonal routine.

Ayurveda also considers periods of your life based on the doshas. From birth to the age of 16 is a Kapha period of growth, 16 to 60 your Pitta period of activity, and 60 onward your Vata period of retirement and inward practices.

Both modern medicine and Ayurveda recommend seeing your doctor, Vaidya, or health expert at least once a year and more if you have any health problems. We also highly recommend you see an integrative health care provider or ayurvedic coach more frequently.

From Biohack to Habit

Let's say you want to improve your daily routine. How can you make this biohack a habit? To complete your Biohack Map and Plan follow the steps below using the graphic.

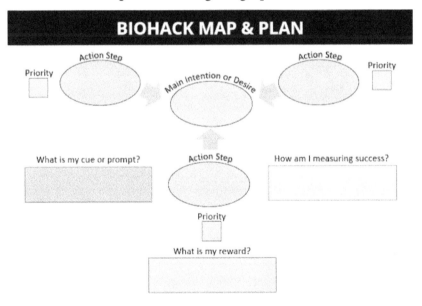

Step 1: Enter your main intention or desire for your biohack in the center.

Step 2: Around the central idea for the biohack enter some

action steps that you think will help accomplish your change.

Step 3: Prioritize your list and choose the main action step that you want to use.

Step 4: Enter a cue or prompt that will help you remember to do your new action step.

Step 5: Determine how you will measure your success with the new biohack and create a reward.

Step 6: Use feedback from self coaching, personal coaching, group coaching, and environmental coaching to keep improving your ability to adopt new habits.

BIOHACK #12

BREATHE

We know that breathing is vital to life and that it helps bring oxygen to all the cells of our body. Today, breathing techniques are being used for relieving stress and anxiety. One of the most popular techniques is diaphragmatic or deep breathing, which involves using the diaphragm muscle to promote relaxation. It is usually done sitting or lying down. Take a slow deep inhalation through your nose. Expand your belly with air and then exhale slowly through your mouth to allow all the air to leave your belly. Place one hand on your chest, which should feel still. Place your other hand on your belly, which should feel the rise and fall with each breath. You can also count while you breathe, with a count of 4 for inhaling, a count of 7 holding the breath, and finally a count of 8 for the gradual exhale.

Breathing techniques have long been important therapeutic strategies in many traditional systems of medicine. In the Vedic Tradition, there is the concept of Prana, the life force that maintains all living things. In the Chinese Taoist tradition there is a similar concept of Chi (or Qi), which is used to describe the vital force that sustains all beings. In both traditions there are many specific breathing techniques and exercises that help regulate the flow of this vital energy throughout the body.

Pranayama

In the Vedic tradition breathing techniques are called pranayama and are often a part of Ayurveda, yoga, and meditation practices. These techniques enhance the connection between mind and body and help to re-establish balance of the doshas. One of the most popular pranayama techniques is called Sukh Pranayama—alternative breathing or Nadi Shodhana Pranayama—which means "channel-cleansing breath." It involves breathing through alternate nostrils. Sit comfortably and cover your right nostril with your thumb, then inhale through the left nostril. Then, close the left nostril with your ring finger and release the thumb from the right nostril and exhale through it. Repeat this process on the other side. This is a simple and effective technique often practiced before meditation practice.

Research shows that our breathing follows regular cycles. These nasal cycles involve the rhythmic switching of the airflow from the right to the left nostril over a period of about 90 minutes. When the airflow is predominantly through the right nostril, higher relative amplitudes of EEG activity are found in the left hemisphere, and vice versa. This balance of dominance can be shifted by intentionally altering the nasal cycle through Pranayama. For example, closing the right nostril and gently breathing through the left nostril causes increased EEG activity in the brain's right hemisphere. The opposite occurs when the nostrils are switched. One study found that changes in EEG patterns occurred almost instantaneously, and after 10 or 15 seconds a long-lasting shift in EEG dominance occurred. These results suggest that by altering the nasal cycle through specific Pranayama exercises, we can alter the neurophysiological functioning of the brain. Incorporating these breathing techniques into your daily routine can help reduce stress and improve your overall health and longevity.

Aromatherapy

Breathing in the aroma of a pure essential oil can have positive effects on health. Studies on essential oils have shown such benefits as reduced anxiety, relief from pain, and enhanced cognitive functions. When we breathe in the volatile molecules of a potent essential oil, they interact with specific olfactory receptors, which then send signals to the brain. Your sense of smell goes straight to your "emotional brain" or limbic system, bypassing the thalamus, which is the normal relay center for the other senses. This is one of the reasons a smell or aroma can often easily evoke a clear and vivid memory or emotion.

There are hundreds of essential oils with different biological actions including natural antibacterial, antifungal, and antiviral properties, as well as analgesic and anti-inflammatory actions. Many studies are currently being done to test all the potential applications of aromatherapy. It is good to note that some people can have an allergic reaction to specific oils, so it is important to test them first and, if possible, take them under the supervision of a qualified aromatherapist.

Quality of Air

The quality of air we breathe is critical for our health and longevity. Poor air quality and pollution can cause health problems such as respiratory disorders, cardiovascular disease, and cancer. Some types of outdoor pollutants include industrial emissions, vehicle exhaust, and wildfires, and these pollutants often have high levels of harmful particles, which can cause respiratory disorders. In addition, there are indoor pollutants such as dust, mold, and chemical emissions that can be responsible for allergies and health problems. Improvements in air quality through filters and other devices can help promote better health and longevity.

From Biohack to Habit

Let's say you want to learn Pranayama. How can you make this biohack a habit? You might want to habit stack by doing your Pranayama right before you meditate. To complete your Biohack Map and Plan follow the steps below using the graphic.

Step 1: Enter your main intention or desire for your biohack in the center.

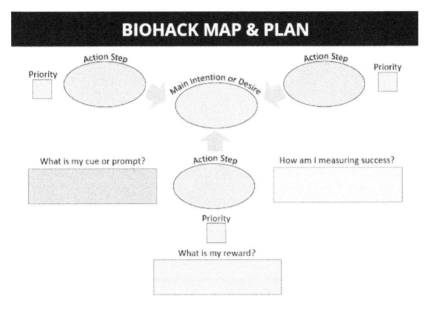

Step 2: Around the central idea for the biohack enter some action steps that you think will help accomplish your change.

Step 3: Prioritize your list and choose the main action step that you want to use.

Step 4: Enter a cue or prompt that will help you remember to do your new action step.

Step 5: Determine how you will measure your success with the new biohack and create a reward.

Step 6: Use from through self coaching, personal coaching, group coaching, and environmental coaching to keep improving your ability to adopt new habits.

BIOHACK #13

WATER

Our bodies are made up of about 60% water, and water is the main component of our blood, which brings nutrients and oxygen to our cells, as well as removing waste products. Water also plays a significant role in temperature regulation, joint activity, digestion, brain function, and healthy skin.

We need to drink enough water to live longer. Recent studies have found a correlation between water balance and muscle strength. Lack of water intake causes dehydration, which can lead to constipation, fatigue, headaches, and kidney problems. With aging there is a loss in the thirst sensation and in the ability to concentrate urine, which can cause cell dehydration and ultimately cell damage.

How much water should we drink? That depends on many factors such as our activity level, age, and gender, as well as the climate. A general guideline is drinking eight glasses of water daily, although not all health experts agree. Water quality is also important since contaminated water can lead to dehydration and serious illnesses such as dysentery, cholera, and typhoid. Our body uses water to help eliminate toxins but if it is contaminated, we are introducing more toxins making it difficult for us to maintain good health. Obviously, there are many types of systems to filter and purify water or you can buy bottled pure water. It is worth a serious investigation.

Ayurveda

The recommendation for the right amount of water according to Ayurveda depends on your predominant dosha or Energy State.

- Vatas need to sip warm water throughout the day in order to stay hydrated. They should try to have a daily intake of about 6-8 cups and avoid drinking too much water at any one time.

- Pittas should have cool or room temperature water and drink 8-10 cups of water daily.

- Kaphas need to drink 8-10 cups of water daily.

It's important to listen to your body and drink water whenever you feel thirsty. Staying properly hydrated is essential for good health, and drinking the right amount of water for your dosha will help support your overall well-being.

Cold-Water Immersion

One of most talked-about biohacks is cold bathing or cold-water immersion, which involves submerging your body in cold water for a short period of time. There is a long history of this practice in the northern countries of Europe. Research suggests that cold bathing may stimulate longevity genes by challenging survival circuits in the body and could have potential health benefits, including improved circulation and immune function, reduced inflammation, and enhanced mood. One published paper reported that regular cold exposure increased lifespan in mice by up to 12%.

It is important to realize that there could be risks for individuals with medical conditions, so it's essential that you consult your healthcare professional before beginning any cold-water immersion on a regular basis.

From Biohack to Habit

Maybe you would like to drink more water each day. How can you make this biohack a habit? To complete your Biohack Map and Plan follow the steps below using the graphic.

Step 1: Enter your main intention or desire for your biohack in the center.

Step 2: Around the central idea for the biohack enter some action steps that you think will help accomplish your change.

Step 3: Prioritize your list and choose the main action step that you want to use.

Step 4: Enter a cue or prompt that will help you remember to do your new action step.

Step 5: Determine how you will measure your success with the new biohack and create a reward.

Step 6: Use feedback from self coaching, personal coaching, group coaching, and environmental coaching to keep improving your ability to adopt new habits.

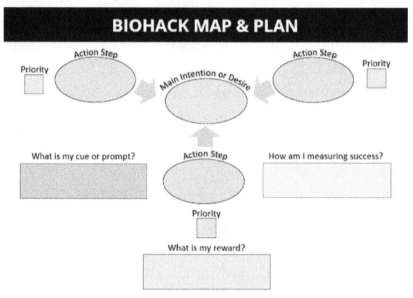

BIOHACK #14

HAPPINESS

Happiness is a key factor for reducing the negative effects of aging because it influences both our physical and mental health. Studies show that older adults who report higher levels of happiness and life satisfaction tend to have better physical health, including lower blood pressure, a stronger immune system, and a reduced risk of heart disease and stroke. Higher levels of happiness and life satisfaction are also correlated with better memory, decision-making abilities, and focus, and even a reduced risk of dementia.

Studies show that older adults who are involved in creative activities such as painting, drawing, or writing, have better health and higher levels of satisfaction, and live longer than those who do not engage in such activities. Also found to be important in individuals who live longer is having a sense of purpose in life and maintaining meaningful social connections and relationships.

The Brain and Happiness

The most basic level of happiness is pleasure or gratification on a physical level. This can come from food, material possessions, entertainment, drugs, alcohol, or sex. It can be short-lived and shallow in nature, and yet powerful enough that many people become addicted to these forms of happiness.

Dopamine is a neurotransmitter that is produced in several parts of our brain, and is involved in different types of behavior, including motivation. In the past, dopamine was associated with happiness, but the latest findings reveal it has more to do with the anticipation of pleasure. It is at the core of most addictions, whether to drugs, food, or social media.

Every time you drink alcohol, play a video game, post a selfie, or smoke a cigarette, you are feeding your dopamine reward network. Key areas in the center of your brain, such as the nucleus accumbens, will become activated as you feed these habits. But your brain resists being overwhelmed and reduces the number of receptors making it harder to turn on the dopamine pathway. As a result, you need more drugs or more cigarettes to feel pleasure. Over a long period of time, addiction changes the functioning of your neural circuits, and the way specific genes are expressed in brain cells.

Dopamine is not the only neurotransmitter associated with happiness. In peak performance, such as winning a race, you get a rush of adrenaline, noradrenaline, and the hormone cortisol. There are also endorphins, which are the body's natural painkillers and are known to be at the basis of a runner's high. Some people become addicted to these moments of achievement, pushing themselves so hard that they become exhausted and stressed.

What about the occasions when we experience joy and love for our partner or our children? This feeling of happiness is at the core of all family life and close bonds, and there is a cocktail of chemicals involved, including dopamine, serotonin, and oxytocin. Serotonin is a "feel-good" neurotransmitter that helps regulate our moods. Oxytocin is a hormone associated with the experience of comfort and love. All of these neurotransmitters and hormones contribute to different forms of happiness.

Scientists are also studying how different neural circuits and areas in the brain interact in moments of happiness. For example, when a person gives something, this can create happiness and it can activate the dopamine reward pathways. There are additional neural circuits involved, for example those responsible for social relationships.

Relationships

One of the most interesting findings in longevity studies is the importance of relationships in both health and longevity. Studies on populations that live longer find that strong relationships are an integral part of the culture of these societies. There is good social support and close relationships between family and friends. Research suggests that social support leads to better physical and mental health. Positive relationships have also been associated with reduced stress and a stronger immune response. Strong relationships give us a sense of purpose and connectedness to the world around us. They help us create beneficial lifestyle choices and increase our overall well-being. Studies also show that loneliness and social isolation can have the opposite effect on our health, weakening our immune response and leading to poor health habits and even addiction.

Ayurveda and Behavioral Rasayanas

There is a section of knowledge in Ayurveda known as behavioral rasayanas, which are types of biohacks to naturally strengthen the body and increase lifespan. Below is a list of some traditional Ayurvedic Behavioral Rasayanas which help improve physiology and health:

- Do everything you can to stay balanced with a good routine.

- Be loving, simple, and compassionate.

- Speak the truth sweetly and uplift others.

- Avoid becoming angry.

- Devote yourself to the knowledge and development of higher states of consciousness.

- Transcend through the regular practice of meditation.

- Be respectful of elders and keep the company
  of the wise.

Ayurveda Guidelines

Ayurveda offers excellent relationship advice based on your Energy State. The following is a summary of some of these recommendations.

V Partner / V Partner

When a balanced V Energy State person is in a relationship with another balanced V partner, the two will probably be very compatible and get joy from each other's creativity. Since both are extremely sensitive, however, if one of them goes out of balance, any slight misunderstanding on either side can cause hurt feelings. If both V Energy State partners go out of balance, life can become an emotional tornado.

Advice:

Both V partners need to stay grounded. V Energy State individuals dislike routines, but the right routine will help to stabilize both their emotions and their physiology, and allow them to be their best selves. V people do not do well in cold and wind and should avoid them as much as possible. (At the very least they need to seriously bundle up in such conditions.) Sipping hot water throughout the day is a simple but powerful way to help balance

V Energy and help prevent illness. Daily warm oil self-massage with a balancing V oil will also help. The master tool for inner and outer balance is, of course, meditation.

P Partner / P Partner

Two P Energy State partners equals fire x 2! But this potentially combustible combination works very well when they are both in good balance because they both have a lot of energy and are highly motivated. They also love competition, physical exercise, and challenges.

Advice:

It is critically important that neither P partner misses a meal or becomes overheated! If either of them goes out of balance, arguments and a power struggle will surely follow. Both people need to understand exactly what triggers a P Energy State outburst. Prevention is key.

K Partner / K Partner

K Energy State partners are like two contented teddy bears. Being on time is never an issue because they have the same slow, steady inner rhythm. If either one of them goes out of balance, however, stubbornness and depression may follow, straining the relationship.

Advice:

K people need to get out, get energized, and interact socially.

This prescription includes a daily dose of active exercise. If, however, both Ks go out of balance, they may need outside help from a coach or trusted friend.

V Partner / P Partner

This can be an amazing relationship. The P Energy State partner is powerful, highly energetic, and driven. The V Energy State partner is sensitive, responsive, and artistic. The hot, fiery P is complemented by the cool, airy V. But when the P person goes out of balance, internal fires can flare out of control and damage the feelings of the more vulnerable V. When they both go out of balance, the relationship may flare and become an emotionally destructive inferno.

Advice:

In this relationship especially, both partners have to focus on staying in good balance. Even then, the P partner must be careful not to be too overbearing or controlling. The V partner has to be careful to stay in balance in order to not become too overly sensitive and emotionally reactive.

V Partner / K Partner

This pair of opposites often makes for an ideal relationship. The calm, easygoing nature of the K partner enjoys and balances the volatile, talkative V partner.

When they both are in good balance, their different operating speeds don't matter. If, however, either one of them goes out of balance, their differences can suddenly result in an argument over trivial things.

Advice:

The V partner is the more sensitive, so the K partner must help the V stay well rested and on a good routine. If the K partner goes out of balance, then the V partner will have to use some energy and strength to help the K get back on track. It is much, much easier for both to take preventive rather than remedial steps to ensure that they stay in balance!

P Partner / K Partner

A P partner in good balance is always motivated toward action and enjoys the challenges of life, while the K partner is calm and capable of handling even the most demanding situations. It is an excellent combination until one of them goes out of balance, and then the situation rapidly falls apart. The P partner will very quickly become intense and controlling, and probably also impatient and angry. The imbalanced K partner is more likely to become withdrawn and stubborn, and difficult to communicate with.

Advice:

Some of the P partner's great energy has to be directed toward helping the K partner continue to be active and in good balance. The natural kindness and steady nature of the K partner must make sure that the P partner eats on time and stays cool!

The Biochemistry of Bliss

Ayurveda speaks about a substance called Ojas, which is considered *the finest product of digestion* in a perfectly healthy digestive system. The more Ojas we have, the stronger our immune system, and the less chance of catching any contagious illness.

Ojas is a more concrete expression of a substance in the Vedic tradition known as Soma, which is a biochemical that allows the experience of bliss in higher states of consciousness, specifically spiritual experiences of the most refined levels of perception.

How can Ojas be identified in terms of modern science? There are many possible candidates for this extraordinary substance. One possibility is serotonin, a key regulator of mood, sleep, appetite, and other brain functions. Your gut produces 90% of all your serotonin, which circulates throughout your bloodstream and influences not only your immune system, but your heart rate, blood clotting, intestinal motility, pulmonary arteries, heart, brain, and mammary glands, as well as the cell growth of liver and bone cells. Another interesting candidate is a chemical called butyric acid, which is produced by the gut bacteria and has numerous beneficial effects, including the improvement of immunity. There are many other possible choices for Ojas, but we will have to wait for conclusive research to finally physically identify this unique ayurvedic substance.

The development of happiness and bliss requires changes on the physical level—changes in neural circuits, changes in the microbiome, and in the levels of hormones and neurotransmitters such as serotonin. One of the reasons the practice of meditation is so important is that we are gradually rebalancing our brain physiology. Every new healthy habit we adopt helps us to replace negative habits with positive ones. Positive health habits help change our brain and microbiome and create the basis for bliss as a permanent part of our daily life.

From Biohack to Habit

Let's say you want to improve your level of happiness. How can you make this biohack a habit? Explore different options for how you make this a habit. To complete your Biohack Map and Plan follow the steps below using the graphic.

Step 1: Enter your main intention or desire for your biohack in the center.

Step 2: Around the central idea for the biohack enter some action steps that you think will help accomplish your change.

Step 3: Prioritize your list and choose the main action step that you want to use.

Step 4: Enter a cue or prompt that will help you remember to do your new action step.

Step 5: Determine how you will measure your success with the new biohack and create a reward.

Step 6: Use feedback from self coaching, personal coaching, group coaching, and environmental coaching to keep improving your ability to adopt new habits.

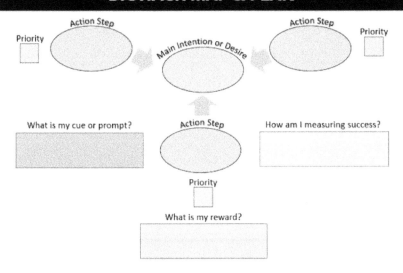

BIOHACK #15

ENVIRONMENT

There are many ways to biohack our environment to live longer. We have considered some of these, such as air and water quality. Other important areas that can affect our health are toxic pesticides, sick building syndrome, and ultimately climate change. Let's focus briefly on some of the things that can be done to improve our environment so that we live long and healthy lives.

Blue Zones

The idea of blue zone communities grew out of research by Gianni Pes and Michel Poulain. They studied the Nuoro province in Sardinia, Italy an area with the largest concentration of centenarian males. Since then, several other locations have been added including Nicoya, Costa Rica; Icaria, Greece; and Okinawa Island, Japan. The people living in these regions tend to eat simple and moderate diets. They exercise regularly, and perhaps most importantly the elderly are treated with respect and as valued members of society.

Any suitable community may be certified as a blue zone and the town I live in, Fairfield, Iowa, was certified in 2015. This was the result of a concentrated effort by community leaders to introduce the world's best practices in food policy, environmental care, exercise opportunities, and social networking. Making it even more supportive, many come twice a day to meditate together in two large domes on the Maharishi International University (MIU) campus with the goal of creating peace for the world. The programs that the university offers are unique in that they combine the ancient knowledge of the Vedic Tradition of India with the most current theories of modern science. In my own department, the Department of Physiology and Health, for example, we offer undergraduate and graduate programs in training health and life coaches in Ayurveda and Integrative Medicine. MIU's College of Integrative Medicine offers a unique fellowship in Integrative Medicine which allows physicians to specialize in Ayurveda. One further interesting consideration is that the buildings on the MIU campus are built according to the Vedic tradition of architecture known as Sthapatya Veda, which is felt to improve the quality of life in a number of different ways.

Collective Consciousness

One of the most interesting concepts in the Vedic Tradition is "collective consciousness." Maharishi Mahesh Yogi explained how this concept could help improve the quality of life everywhere.

According to the Vedic Tradition, consciousness is not merely an individual condition, but rather it is a unified field which underlies all mind and matter. We are familiar with fields of electromagnetic radiation, radio waves, and X-rays, but typically we do not think of consciousness as a field.

Maharishi explained that we can influence the "collective consciousness"—the sum of the consciousness of all the people in a society—in a positive way through the group practice of Transcendental Meditation and its advanced programs. There is a phrase in the Yoga Sutras of Patanjali to which Maharishi often refers: "In the vicinity of yoga all hostile tendencies disappear." Practically speaking what this means is that the coherence created in the brain of each individual during their practice of Transcendental Meditation and its advanced programs influences the collective consciousness of their society and produces a positive influence in the behavior of others even those who are not meditating.

Over 30 peer-reviewed scientific studies have demonstrated the fact that the TM technique can be used as a technology to create a positive effect on the behavior of a given society. These remarkable results have been published in such journals as: *Journal of Conflict Resolution, Journal of Social Behavior and Personality, The Journal of Mind and Behavior, Social Indicators Research,* and *Psychology, Crime & Law.* The studies show that when groups of practitioners of Transcendental Meditation and its advanced programs meditate together, there is a measurable decrease in violence and an increase in positive trends in society. This phenomenon has been appropriately named the "Maharishi Effect" since it was predicted by Maharishi many years ago. This is perhaps the most powerful biohack in the world. Improve the quality of life by creating coherence in the collective consciousness, and we will all live longer.

From Biohack to Habit

Let's say you want to improve your environment. How can you make this biohack a habit? To complete your Biohack Map and Plan follow the steps below using the graphic.

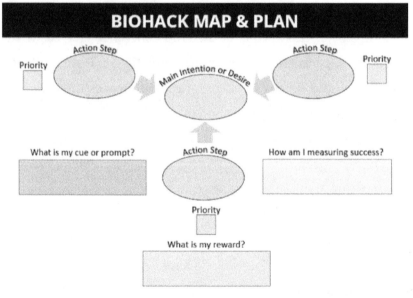

Step 1: Enter your main intention or desire for your biohack in the center.

Step 2: Around the central idea for the biohack enter some action steps that you think will help accomplish your change.

Step 3: Prioritize your list and choose the main action step that you want to use.

Step 4: Enter a cue or prompt that will help you remember to do your new action step.

Step 5: Determine how you will measure your success with the new biohack and create a reward.

Step 6: Use feedback from self coaching, personal coaching, group coaching, and environmental coaching to keep improving your ability to adopt new habits.

BIOHACK #16

SPIRITUALITY

Spirituality can have a significant impact on our health and longevity. There are many possible definitions of spirituality, ranging from a belief in God as part of an established religion, to recognizing that there is something greater than ourselves, to an appreciation of the cosmic, sacred, and divine in nature and in everyone and everything around us.

Studies show a correlation between more positive beliefs and better physical health. Spirituality provides social support, a sense of purpose, and an appreciation of community. All of these elements improve mental and physical health, especially as people get older and face the concept of death.

The Placebo Effect

We have finally learned that there is an intimate connection between the mind and body. Research on the placebo effect reveals that it is possible for belief to directly affect our health. The placebo effect has been defined as an improvement in health caused by an intervention that has no direct physical-chemical effect on the ailment. Studies have shown that the placebo effect is associated with significant improvement in many health conditions, including pain, depression, anxiety, and irritable bowel syndrome. Neuroimaging studies identify specific brain areas involved in the placebo effect and specific neurotransmitters responsible for this phenomenon. One study found that the placebo effect accounted for up to 75% of the positive response to antidepressant medications. People taking a placebo pill often experienced the same level of improvement in symptoms as those taking the medication.

Dr. Alia Crum of Stanford University argues that mindset is the key to the placebo effect. In one study, Dr. Crum and her collaborators investigated the concept that a nutritional label could physically change what happens to you. She gave subjects two milkshakes a week apart. One vanilla milkshake was called Sensishake and was said to have zero percent fat, zero added sugar, and only 140 calories. The second milkshake was called Indulgence and according to its label, had enough sugar and fat to account for 620 calories. In fact, both shakes had 300 calories each. Before and after taking the milkshakes, measurements were made on the levels of the hormone ghrelin. Ghrelin is secreted in the gut and has been called the "hunger" hormone because levels rise when you are hungry. In her study, Dr. Crum found that ghrelin levels dropped about three times more when people were consuming the indulgent shake compared to the people who drank the sensible shake. The study suggests that the belief of subjects who drank the indulgent shake influenced their body to think it was more full.

What these and other studies indicate is that a healthier mindset helps to create a healthier body. Further studies have emphasized the need for healthcare providers to implement better bedside manners. You may not be able to think yourself into living a longer life but a growth mindset may well give you a better chance.

Spirituality and Consciousness

Does spirituality require us to believe in God or can we take a scientific view? For Einstein, these concepts were the same.

> My religion consists of a humble admiration of the illimitable superior spirit who reveals himself in the slight details we are able to perceive with our frail and feeble minds. That deeply emotional conviction of the presence of a superior reasoning power, which is revealed in the incomprehensible universe, forms my idea of God. —Albert Einstein

The ancient Greeks had their own expression of the connection between the individual and cosmos.

> You ask, how can we know the Infinite? I answer, not by reason….You can only apprehend the Infinite… by entering into a state in which you are finite self no longer, in which the divine essence is communicated

to you. This is Ecstasy. It is the liberation of your mind
from its finite consciousness. Like only can apprehend
like; when you thus cease to finite, you become one with
the Infinite. In the reunion of your soul to its simplest
self, its divine essence, you realize this Union—this
Identity. —Plotinus

One of the greatest contributions to the understanding of consciousness is the research of Tony Nader, M.D., Ph.D., a graduate
of MIT and Harvard, who worked intensively with Maharishi
Mahesh Yogi to reveal the relationship between human physiology and the details of the Vedic literature. In his first book *Human
Physiology: Expression of Veda and the Vedic Literature*, Dr Nader
shows that the order of Veda and the Vedic literature is mirrored
in the intrinsic order of human physiology. The idea is that the
outer macrocosm of natural law is mapped within the inner mi-
crocosm of our physiology.

In his second book, *Ramayan in Human Physiology*, Dr. Nader
unfolds even more detailed correlations focusing on the story of
the Ramayan, a beloved pillar of Indian culture. The Ramayan is
at once a spiritual story about an avatar, an incarnation of God,
a story of perfect rulership and administration, and on the epic
heroic tale that portrays the full range of human emotion. Like
the Greek tale of Ulysses and other classic myths, it is the story
of a hero who must embark upon a journey and undergo many
challenges, ultimately conquering a terrible demon and returning
home victorious.

The eminent scholar Joseph Campbell painstakingly researched some of the greatest hero epics of all cultures and located certain common features or archetypes occurring in each of them. Campbell tells us that these stories serve as a metaphor for the individual psychological development of every human being. The journeys of the heroes are symbolic of our natural search for truth and enlightenment, while their return home symbolizes the realization that everything we most deeply desire lies in our own heart and brain.

Dr. Nader's work postulates that the hero's journey is not merely psychological, but is an actual description of the neurophysiological mechanisms involved in gaining enlightenment. Rather than describing physical transformations in today's scientific terms, the creators of these stories used the language of myth and poetry. The hero's final victory is the slaying of a demon, which symbolizes the removal of some huge abnormality or stress in the body that supports destructive behavior. This process is accomplished by creating coherent neural networks which enable us to realize our fullest mental and emotional potential.

The significance of Dr. Nader's work is that we can now understand that the ancient hero myths of world culture and religion describe a universal process of spiritual realization, a process that involves highly specific changes in human brain functioning. Whatever the language, the message is the same—the journey of the hero is the journey of finding our inner Self.

Let the eye of your heart be opened that you may see the spirit and behold invisible things….You will journey beyond the narrow limitations of time and place and thence you will pass into the infinite space of the Divine World. What ear hath not heard, that you will hear, and what no eye hath seen, you shall behold: until you shall be brought to the high Abode, where you will see One only, out of the world and all worldly creatures. To that One you shall devote the love of both heart and soul, until with the eye that knows no doubt, you will see plainly that One is and there is nothing save Him alone: there is no God save Him. —Hatif of Isfahan, Sufi Seer

Vedic Sound

One of the interesting applications of Dr. Nader's discovery is Vedic Sound Therapy. Many ancient natural systems of medicine used sounds to help restore balance in the physiology. Dr. Hari Sharma at Ohio State University found experimental evidence suggesting that the sounds of the Vedic literature have a beneficial effect on re-enlivening the inner intelligence of the cell. The effects of Vedic sounds were compared to that of hard rock music and a no-sound condition on the growth of cells in culture. Five types of human cancer cells (lung, colon, brain, breast, and melanoma) and one normal cell type were tested in four experiments. The recordings of Vedic sounds and hard rock were adjusted so that the degree of loudness was similar for both. The Vedic sounds decreased growth in all of the cancer cell types. In the presence of hard rock music, cancer cell growth was generally increased, although effects were not consistent.

Listening to Vedic Sounds resets the sequential unfoldment of intelligence in our body to match its original pattern, and thus removes any physiological imbalances. As the impulses of sound reverberate in the awareness, a kind of sympathetic resonance occurs; they act as a template that can restore the body to a state of balance.

Dr. Nader's latest book, *One Unbounded Ocean of Consciousness,* gives us a comprehensive understanding of the relationship between the latest discoveries of modern science and the ancient Vedic understanding of Unity Consciousness. How we see the world depends upon our state of consciousness, which in turn depends upon the state of our nervous system. The ultimate level of spirituality is the reality of a nervous system so refined that we can directly experience the unified field of all the laws of nature.

Karma and Free Will

Karma is the ancient concept. It describes a person's actions, thoughts, and intentions have consequences that determine their future experiences, both in this life and in the future lives or incarnations. In some cultures, karma is taken to be the ultimate factor which determines how long you live. One's life is measured by a contract of a specific number of breaths. Yet karma does not rule free will.

According to this perspective, we can shorten our life by

expending our breaths quickly or we can extend it by creating a more efficient physiology that lowers our breath rate while we are still active. The choice is our own. Rather than leave our lives to fate or karma, it is important that we take responsibility for our choices, because ultimately they will determine our health and longevity. If we chose bad health habits, we are far more likely to be unhealthy and live a shorter life. To be healthy and live a long life we want to make positive choices, which are often based on our core beliefs. The most important belief is in yourself—that you can improve and empower yourself to unfold your full potential. This is the greatest of all biohacks and it is present within each one of us.

ABOUT THE AUTHORS

DR. ROBERT KEITH WALLACE

Dr. Robert Keith Wallace did pioneering research on the Transcendental Meditation technique. His seminal papers—published in *Science, American Journal of Physiology,* and *Scientific American*—on a fourth major state of consciousness support a new paradigm of mind-body medicine and total brain development. Dr. Wallace is the founding President of Maharishi International University, has traveled around the world giving lectures at major universities and institutes, and has written and co-authored many books.

He is presently a Trustee of Maharishi International University and Chairman of the Department of Physiology and Health.

TED WALLACE

Ted Wallace is currently an Agile Coach at Principal Financial Group. He has completed two Master of Science degrees, one in Computer Science and the other in Physiology, at Maharishi International University. He is a certified Scrum Master Professional (CSM, CSPO, CSP, CTC) and a registered corporate coach (RCC) with thousands of hours of coaching sessions.

SAMANTHA WALLACE

A former model, Samantha Jones Wallace was featured on the covers of such magazines as *Vogue, Cosmopolitan, Good Housekeeping,* and *Look.* She is a long-time practitioner of Transcendental Meditation and has a deep understanding of Ayurveda and its relationship to health and well-being. Samantha is a co-author of *Gut Crisis, The Rest And Repair Diet, The Coherence Code, Total Brain Coaching,* and *Trouble In Paradise.*

She is also the co-author of *Quantum Golf* (Editions One and Two) and was an editor of *Dharma Parenting.* Happily married for over forty years, the Wallaces have a combined family of four children and six grandchildren.

ACKNOWLEDGMENTS

Our deep appreciation goes to our very talented friends—George Foster for his outstanding cover design and Carol Paredes and Allen Cobb for their help with graphics.

We would also like to thank Joel Silver, Carol Paredes, Fran Clark, and Nicole Windenberger for excellent sugggestions, editing, and proofreading.

R E F E R E N C E S

USEFUL WEBSITES

biohacklongevity.com

TM.org

MIU.edu

USEFUL REFERENCES

Introduction

Heterochronic parabiosis: historical perspective and methodological considerations for studies of aging and longevity. Aging Cell. 2013 Jun;12(3):525-30. doi: 10.1111/acel.12065. Epub 2013 Apr 10. PMID: 23489470; PMCID: PMC4072458.

Pálovics R, Keller A, Schaum N, Tan W, Fehlmann T, Borja M, Kern F, Bonanno L, Calcuttawala K, Webber J, McGeever A; Tabula Muris Consortium, Luo J, Pisco AO, Karkanias J, Neff NF, Darmanis S, Quake SR, Wyss-Coray T. Molecular hallmarks of heterochronic parabiosis at single-cell resolution. Nature. 2022 Mar;603(7900):309-314. doi: 10.1038/s41586-022-04461-2. Epub 2022 Mar 2. PMID: 35236985; PM-CID: PMC9387403.

Yang C, Liu ZL, Wang J, Bu XL, Wang YJ, Xiang Y. Parabiosis modeling:

protocol, application and perspectives. Zool Res. 2021 May 18;42(3):253-261. doi: 10.24272/j.issn.2095-8137.2020.368. PMID: 33723928; PMCID: PMC8175960.

Hofmann B. Young Blood Rejuvenates Old Bodies: A Call for Reflection when Moving from Mice to Men. Transfus Med Hemother. 2018 Jan;45(1):67-71. doi: 10.1159/000481828. Epub 2018 Jan 3. PMID: 29593463; PMCID: PMC5836258.

Buettner D, Skemp S. Blue Zones: Lessons From the World's Longest Lived. Am J Lifestyle Med. 2016 Jul 7;10(5):318-321. doi: 10.1177/1559827616637066. PMID: 30202288; PMCID: PMC6125071.

Pálovics R, Keller A, Schaum N, Tan W, Fehlmann T, Borja M, Kern F, Bonanno L, Calcuttawala K, Webber J, McGeever A; Tabula Muris Consortium, Luo J, Pisco AO, Karkanias J, Neff NF, Darmanis S, Quake SR, Wyss-Coray T. Molecular hallmarks of heterochronic parabiosis at single-cell resolution. Nature. 2022 Mar;603(7900):309-314. doi: 10.1038/s41586-022-04461-2. Epub 2022 Mar 2. PMID: 35236985; PMCID: PMC9387403.

Conboy MJ, Conboy IM, Rando TA. Heterochronic parabiosis: historical perspective and methodological considerations for studies of aging and longevity. Aging Cell. 2013 Jun;12(3):525-30. doi: 10.1111/acel.12065. Epub 2013 Apr 10. PMID: 23489470; PMCID: PMC4072458.

Pifferi F, Terrien J, Marchal J, Dal-Pan A, Djelti F, Hardy I, Chahory S, Cordonnier N, Desquilbet L, Hurion M, Zahariev A, Chery I, Zizzari P, Perret M, Epelbaum J, Blanc S, Picq JL, Dhenain M, Aujard F. Caloric restriction increases lifespan but affects brain integrity in grey mouse lemur primates. Commun Biol. 2018 Apr 5;1:30. doi: 10.1038/s42003-018-0024-8. PMID: 30271916; PMCID: PMC6123706.

Yankova T, Dubiley T, Shytikov D, Pishel I. Three Month Heterochronic Parabiosis Has a Deleterious Effect on the Lifespan of Young Animals, Without a Positive Effect for Old Animals. Rejuvenation Res. 2022 Aug;25(4):191-199. doi: 10.1089/rej.2022.0029. Epub 2022 Jul 22. PMID: 35747947.

Pal S, Tyler JK. Epigenetics and aging. Sci Adv. 2016 Jul 29;2(7):e1600584. doi: 10.1126/sciadv.1600584. PMID: 27482540; PMCID: PMC4966880.

Wątroba M, Dudek I, Skoda M, Stangret A, Rzodkiewicz P, Szukiewicz

D. Sirtuins, epigenetics and longevity. Ageing Res Rev. 2017 Nov;40:11-19. doi: 10.1016/j.arr.2017.08.001. Epub 2017 Aug 5. PMID: 28789901.

Salehi B, Stojanović-Radić Z, Matejić J, Sharifi-Rad M, Anil Kumar NV, Martins N, Sharifi-Rad J. The therapeutic potential of curcumin: A review of clinical trials. Eur J Med Chem. 2019 Feb 1;163:527-545. doi: 10.1016/j.ejmech.2018.12.016. Epub 2018 Dec 7. PMID: 30553144.

Nelson KM, Dahlin JL, Bisson J, Graham J, Pauli GF, Walters MA. The Essential Medicinal Chemistry of Curcumin. J Med Chem. 2017 Mar 9;60(5):1620-1637. doi: 10.1021/acs.jmedchem.6b00975. Epub 2017 Jan 11. PMID: 28074653; PMCID: PMC5346970.

Biohack #1

Atomic Habits: An Easy & Proven Way to Build Good Habits & Break Bad Ones by James Clear, Avery, 2018

Tiny Habits: The Small Changes That Change Everything by BJ Fogg, Houghton Mifflin Harcourt, 2019

The Power of Habit: Why We Do What We Do in Life and Business by Charles Duhigg, Random House, 2012

The Rest And Repair Diet: Heal Your Gut, Improve Your Physical and Mental Health, and Lose Weight by Robert Keith Wallace, PhD, Samantha Wallace, Andrew Stenberg, MA, Jim Davis, DO, and Alexis Farley, Dharma Publications, 2019

Total Brain Coaching: A Holistic System of Effective Habit Change For the Individual, Team, and Organization by Ted Wallace, MS, Robert Keith Wallace, PhD, and Samantha Wallace, Dharma Publications, 2020

Self Empower: Using Self Coaching, Neuroadaptability, and Ayurveda by Robert Keith Wallace, PhD, Samantha Wallace, Ted Wallace, MS, Dharma Publications, 2021

Wallace, R.K.; Wallace, T. Neuroadaptability and Habit: Modern Medicine and Ayurveda. Medicina 2021, 57, 90. doi: 10.3390/medicina57020090

Biohack #2

Travis FT and Shear J. Focused attention, open monitoring and automatic self-transcending: Categories to organize meditations from Vedic, Buddhist and Chinese traditions. Consciousness and Cognition 19(4):1110-1118, 2010

Wallace RK. Physiological effects of Transcendental Meditation. Science 167:1751-1754, 1970

Wallace RK, et al. A wakeful hypometabolic physiologic state. American Journal of Physiology 221(3): 795-799, 1971

Wallace RK. Physiological effects of the Transcendental Meditation technique: A proposed fourth major state of consciousness. Ph.D. thesis. Physiology Department, University of California, Los Angeles, 1970

Schneider RH, et al. Stress Reduction in the Secondary Prevention of Cardiovascular Disease: Randomized, Controlled Trial of Transcendental Meditation and Health Education in Blacks. Circ Cardiovasc Qual Outcomes 5:750-758, 2012

Rainforth MV, et al. Stress reduction programs in patients with elevated blood pressure: a systematic review and meta-analysis. Current Hypertension Reports 9:520–528, 2007

Brook RD, et al. Beyond Medications and Diet: Alternative Approaches to Lowering Blood Pressure. A Scientific Statement from the American Heart Association. Hypertension 61(6):1360-83, 2013

Cooper MJ, et al. Transcendental Meditation in the management of hypercholesterolemia. Journal of Human Stress 5(4): 24–27, 1979

Orme-Johnson DW and Walton KW. All approaches of preventing or reversing effects of stress are not the same. American Journal of Health Promotion 12:297-299, 1998

Barnes VA, et al. Impact of Transcendental Meditation on cardiovascular function at rest and during acute stress in adolescents with high normal blood pressure. Journal of Psychosomatic Research 51: 597-605, 2001

Jevning R, et al. Adrenocortical activity during meditation. Hormonal Behavior 10(1):54-60, 1978

Paul-Labrador M, et al. Effects of randomized controlled trial of Transcendental Meditation on components of the metabolic syndrome in subjects with coronary heart disease. Archives of Internal Medicine 166:1218-1224, 2006

Alexander CN, et al. Treating and preventing alcohol, nicotine, and drug abuse through Transcendental Meditation: A review and statistical meta-analysis. Alcoholism Treatment Quarterly 11: 13-87, 1994

Orme-Johnson DW, Herron RE. An Innovative Approach to Reducing Medical Care Utilization and Expenditures. American Journal of Managed Care 3: 135–144, 1997

Herron RE. Can the Transcendental Meditation Program Reduce the Medical Expenditures of Older People? A Longitudinal Cost-Reduction Study in Canada. Journal of Social Behavior and Personality 17(1): 415–442, 2005

Wallace RK, et al. The effects of the Transcendental Meditation and TM-Sidhi program on the aging process. International Journal of Neuroscience 16: 53-58, 1982

Glaser JL, Brind JL, Vogelman JH, Eisner MJ, Dillbeck MC, Wallace RK, Chopra D, Orentreich N. Elevated serum dehydroepiandrosterone sulfate levels in practitioners of the Transcendental Meditation (TM) and TM-Sidhi programs. J Behav Med. 1992 Aug;15(4):327-41. doi: 10.1007/BF00844726. PMID: 1404349.

Alexander CN, et al. Transcendental Meditation, mindfulness, and longevity. Journal of Personality and Social Psychology 57: 950-964, 1989

Alexander CN, et al. The effects of Transcendental Meditation compared to other methods of relaxation in reducing risk factors, morbidity, and mortality. Homeostasis 35: 243-264, 1994

Schneider RH, et al. Long-term effects of stress reduction on mortality in persons > 55 years of age with systemic hypertension. American Journal of Cardiology 95: 1060-1064, 2005

Duraimani S, et al. Effects of Lifestyle Modification on Telomerase Gene Expression in Hypertensive Patients: A Pilot Trial of Stress Reduction and Health Education Programs in African Americans. PLOS ONE 10(11): e0142689, 2015

Wenuganen S, Walton KG, Katta S, Dalgard CL, Sukumar G, Starr J,

Travis FT, Wallace RK, Morehead P, Lonsdorf NK, Srivastava M, Fagan J. Transcriptomics of Long-Term Meditation Practice: Evidence for Prevention or Reversal of Stress Effects Harmful to Health. Medicina (Kaunas) 57(3): 218, 2021

Alexander CN, et al. Transcendental Meditation, self-actualization, and psychological health: A conceptual overview and statistical meta-analysis. Journal of Social Behavior and Personality 6: 189-247, 1991

Eppley KR, et al. Differential effects of relaxation techniques on trait anxiety: A meta-analysis. Journal of Clinical Psychology 45: 957-974, 1989

Alexander CN, et al. Effects of the Transcendental Meditation program on stress-reduction, health, and employee development: A prospective study in two occupational settings. Stress, Anxiety and Coping 6: 245–262, 1993

Harung HS, et al. Peak performance and higher states of consciousness: A study of world-class performers. Journal of Managerial Psychology 11(4): 3–23, 1996

Nidich S, et al. Non-trauma-focused meditation versus exposure therapy in veterans with post-traumatic stress disorder: a randomised controlled trial. Lancet Psychiatry 5(12):975-986, 2018

Wallace RK, Wallace T. Neuroadaptability and Habit: Modern Medicine and Ayurveda. Medicina (Kaunas). 2021 Jan 21;57(2):90. doi: 10.3390/medicina57020090. PMID: 33494269; PMCID: PMC7909780.

Biohack #3

Hamblin MR. Photobiomodulation for Alzheimer's Disease: Has the Light Dawned? Photonics. 2019 Sep;6(3):77. doi: 10.3390/photonics6030077. Epub 2019 Jul 4. PMID: 31363464; PMCID: PMC6664299.

Montazeri K, Farhadi M, Fekrazad R, Akbarnejad Z, Chaibakhsh S, Mahmoudian S. Transcranial photobiomodulation in the management of brain disorders. J Photochem Photobiol B. 2021 Aug;221:112207. doi: 10.1016/j.jphotobiol.2021.112207. Epub 2021 May 5. PMID: 34119804.

Do MTH. Melanopsin and the Intrinsically Photosensitive

Retinal Ganglion Cells: Biophysics to Behavior. Neuron. 2019 Oct 23;104(2):205-226. doi: 10.1016/j.neuron.2019.07.016. PMID: 31647894; PMCID: PMC6944442.

Lazzerini Ospri L, Prusky G, Hattar S. Mood, the Circadian System, and Melanopsin Retinal Ganglion Cells. Annu Rev Neurosci. 2017 Jul 25;40:539-556. doi: 10.1146/annurev-neuro-072116-031324. Epub 2017 May 17. PMID: 28525301; PMCID: PMC5654534.

Barolet D, Christiaens F, Hamblin MR. Infrared and skin: Friend or foe. J Photochem Photobiol B. 2016 Feb;155:78-85. doi: 10.1016/j.jphotobiol.2015.12.014. Epub 2015 Dec 21. PMID: 26745730; PMCID: PMC4745411

Reiter RJ, Tan DX, Rosales-Corral S, Galano A, Zhou XJ, Xu B. Mitochondria: Central Organelles for Melatonin's Antioxidant and Anti-Aging Actions. Molecules. 2018 Feb 24;23(2):509. doi: 10.3390/molecules 23020509. PMID: 29495303; PMCID: PMC6017324.

Reiter RJ, Ma Q, Sharma R. Melatonin in Mitochondria: Mitigating Clear and Present Dangers. Physiology (Bethesda). 2020 Mar 1;35(2):86-95. doi: 10.1152/physiol.00034.2019. PMID: 32024428.

Melhuish Beaupre LM, Brown GM, Gonçalves VF, Kennedy JL. Melatonin's neuroprotective role in mitochondria and its potential as a biomarker in aging, cognition and psychiatric disorders. Transl Psychiatry. 2021 Jun 2;11(1):339. doi: 10.1038/s41398-021-01464-x. PMID: 34078880; PMCID: PMC8172874.

Reiter RJ, Sharma R, Pires de Campos Zuccari DA, de Almeida Chuffa LG, Manucha W, Rodriguez C. Melatonin synthesis in and uptake by mitochondria: implications for diseased cells with dysfunctional mitochondria. Future Med Chem. 2021 Feb;13(4):335-339. doi: 10.4155/fmc-2020-0326. Epub 2021 Jan 5. PMID: 33399498.

Engel KW, Khan I, Arany PR. Cell lineage responses to photobiomodulation therapy. J Biophotonics. 2016 Dec;9(11-12):1148-1156. doi: 10.1002/jbio.201600025. Epub 2016 Jul 8. PMID: 27392170.

Srivastava AK, Roy Choudhury S, Karmakar S. Near-Infrared Responsive Dopamine/Melatonin-Derived Nanocomposites Abrogating in Situ Amyloid β Nucleation, Propagation, and Ameliorate Neuronal Functions. ACS Appl Mater Interfaces. 2020 Feb 5;12(5):5658-5670. doi:

10.1021/acsami.9b22214. Epub 2020 Jan 27. PMID: 31986005.

Reiter RJ, Sharma R, Rosales-Corral S. Anti-Warburg Effect of Melatonin: A Proposed Mechanism to Explain its Inhibition of Multiple Diseases. Int J Mol Sci. 2021 Jan 14;22(2):764. doi: 10.3390/ijms22020764. PMID: 33466614; PMCID: PMC7828708.

Dr Andrew Huberman, Neurobiologicist and Associate Professor at Stanford talks about the value of sunlight: https://www.youtube.com/watch?v=yBjUR16AiBMD

Biohack #4

Lifespan: Why We Age—and Why We Don't Have To by David Sinclair and Matthew LaPlante, Atria Books; Illustrated edition 2019

Cho Y, Hong N, Kim KW, Cho SJ, Lee M, Lee YH, Lee YH, Kang ES, Cha BS, Lee BW. The Effectiveness of Intermittent Fasting to Reduce Body Mass Index and Glucose Metabolism: A Systematic Review and Meta-Analysis. J Clin Med. 2019 Oct 9;8(10):1645. doi: 10.3390/jcm8101645. PMID: 31601019; PMCID: PMC6832593.

Longo VD, Mattson MP. Fasting: molecular mechanisms and clinical applications. Cell Metab. 2014 Feb 4;19(2):181-92. doi: 10.1016/j.cmet.2013.12.008. Epub 2014 Jan 16. PMID: 24440038; PMCID: PMC3946160

Welton S, Minty R, O'Driscoll T, Willms H, Poirier D, Madden S, Kelly L. Intermittent fasting and weight loss: Systematic review. Can Fam Physician. 2020 Feb;66(2):117-125. PMID: 32060194; PMCID: PMC7021351.

Dong TA, Sandesara PB, Dhindsa DS, Mehta A, Arneson LC, Dollar AL, Taub PR, Sperling LS. Intermittent Fasting: A Heart Healthy Dietary Pattern? Am J Med. 2020 Aug;133(8):901-907. doi: 10.1016/j.amjmed.2020.03.030. Epub 2020 Apr 21. PMID: 32330491; PMCID: PMC7415631

Allaf M, Elghazaly H, Mohamed OG, Fareen MFK, Zaman S, Salmasi AM, Tsilidis K, Dehghan A. Intermittent fasting for the prevention of cardiovascular disease. Cochrane Database Syst Rev. 2021 Jan 29;1(1):CD013496. doi: 10.1002/14651858.CD013496.pub2. PMID:

33512717; PMCID: PMC8092432.

Hammer SS, Vieira CP, McFarland D, Sandler M, Levitsky Y, Dorweiler TF, Lydic TA, Asare-Bediako B, Adu-Agyeiwaah Y, Sielski MS, Dupont M, Longhini AL, Li Calzi S, Chakraborty D, Seigel GM, Proshlyakov DA, Grant MB, Busik JV. Fasting and fasting-mimicking treatment activate SIRT1/LXRα and alleviate diabetes-induced systemic and microvascular dysfunction. Diabetologia. 2021 Jul;64(7):1674-1689. doi: 10.1007/s00125-021-05431-5. Epub 2021 Mar 26. PMID: 33770194; PMCID: PMC8236268.

Lingappa N, Mayrovitz H N (September 04, 2022) Role of Sirtuins in Diabetes and Age-Related Processes. Cureus 14(9): e28774. doi:10.7759/cureus.28774

Gut Crisis: How Diet, Probiotics, and Friendly Bacteria Help You Lose Weight and Heal Your Body and Mind by Robert Keith Wallace, PhD, Samantha Wallace, Dharma Publications, 2017

The Rest And Repair Diet: Heal Your Gut, Improve Your Physical and Mental Health, and Lose Weight by Robert Keith Wallace, PhD, Samantha Wallace, Andrew Sternberg, MA Jim Davis, DO, and Alexis Farley, Dharma Publications, 2019

Biohack #5

Vitamin B12

Green R, Allen LH, Bjørke-Monsen AL, Brito A, Guéant JL, Miller JW, Molloy AM, Nexo E, Stabler S, Toh BH, Ueland PM, Yajnik C. Vitamin B12 deficiency. Nat Rev Dis Primers. 2017 Jun 29;3:17040. doi: 10.1038/nrdp.2017.40. Erratum in: Nat Rev Dis Primers. 2017 Jul 20;3:17054. PMID: 28660890.

Gana W, De Luca A, Debacq C, Poitau F, Poupin P, Aidoud A, Fougère B. Analysis of the Impact of Selected Vitamins Deficiencies on the Risk of Disability in Older People. Nutrients. 2021 Sep 10;13(9):3163. doi: 10.3390/nu13093163. PMID: 34579039; PMCID: PMC8469089.

Vitamin D

Gana W, De Luca A, Debacq C, Poitau F, Poupin P, Aidoud A, Fougère B. Analysis of the Impact of Selected Vitamins Deficiencies on the Risk of Disability in Older People. Nutrients. 2021 Sep 10;13(9):3163. doi: 10.3390/nu13093163. PMID: 34579039; PMCID: PMC8469089.

Roth DE, Abrams SA, Aloia J, Bergeron G, Bourassa MW, Brown KH, Calvo MS, Cashman KD, Combs G, De-Regil LM, Jefferds ME, Jones KS, Kapner H, Martineau AR, Neufeld LM, Schleicher RL, Thacher TD, Whiting SJ. Global prevalence and disease burden of vitamin D deficiency: a roadmap for action in low- and middle-income countries. Ann N Y Acad Sci. 2018 Oct;1430(1):44-79. doi: 10.1111/nyas.13968. Epub 2018 Sep 18. PMID: 30225965; PMCID: PMC7309365.

Touvier M, Deschasaux M, Montourcy M, Sutton A, Charnaux N, Kesse-Guyot E, Assmann KE, Fezeu L, Latino-Martel P, Druesne-Pecollo N, Guinot C, Latreille J, Malvy D, Galan P, Hercberg S, Le Clerc S, Souberbielle JC, Ezzedine K. Determinants of vitamin D status in Caucasian adults: influence of sun exposure, dietary intake, sociodemographic, lifestyle, anthropometric, and genetic factors. J Invest Dermatol. 2015 Feb;135(2):378-388. doi: 10.1038/jid.2014.400. Epub 2014 Sep 11. PMID: 25211176.

Vitamin C

Hemilä H, Chalker E. Vitamin C for preventing and treating the common cold. Cochrane Database Syst Rev. 2013 Jan 31;2013(1):CD000980. doi: 10.1002/14651858.CD000980.pub4. PMID: 23440782; PMCID: PMC8078152.

Hemilä H. Vitamin C and Infections. Nutrients. 2017 Mar 29;9(4):339. doi: 10.3390/nu9040339. PMID: 28353648; PMCID: PMC5409678.

Travica N, Ried K, Sali A, Hudson I, Scholey A, Pipingas A. Plasma Vitamin C Concentrations and Cognitive Function: A Cross-Sectional Study. Front Aging Neurosci. 2019 Apr 2;11:72. doi: 10.3389/fnagi.2019.00072. PMID: 31001107; PMCID: PMC6454201.

Pham-Huy LA, He H, Pham-Huy C. Free radicals, antioxidants in disease and health. Int J Biomed Sci. 2008 Jun;4(2):89-96. PMID: 23675073; PMCID: PMC3614697.

Kim MK, Sasazuki S, Sasaki S, Okubo S, Hayashi M, Tsugane S. Effect of five-year supplementation of vitamin C on serum vitamin C concentration and consumption of vegetables and fruits in middle-aged Japanese: a randomized controlled trial. J Am Coll Nutr. 2003 Jun;22(3):208-16. doi: 10.1080/07315724.2003.10719295. PMID: 12805247.

Zinc

Hou R, He Y, Yan G, Hou S, Xie Z, Liao C. Zinc enzymes in medicinal chemistry. Eur J Med Chem. 2021 Dec 15;226:113877. doi: 10.1016/j.ejmech.2021.113877. Epub 2021 Sep 30. PMID: 34624823.

Prasad, Ananda S.: "Discovery of Human Zinc Deficiency: Its Impact on Human Health and Disease", March 6 2013, ncbi.nlm.nih.gov/pmc/articles/PMC3649098/

Afzali A, Goli S, Moravveji A, Bagheri H, Mirhosseini S, Ebrahimi H. The effect of zinc supplementation on fatigue among elderly community dwellers: A parallel clinical trial. Health Sci Rep. 2021 May 19;4(2):e301. doi: 10.1002/hsr2.301. PMID: 34027128; PMCID: PMC8133867.

Multivitamins

Moyer VA, U. S. Preventive Services Task Force. Vitamin, mineral, and multivitamin supplements for the primary prevention of cardiovascular disease and cancer: U.S. Preventive services Task Force recommendation statement. Ann Intern Med. 2014;160(8):558–64. PMID: 24566474. 10.7326/M14-0198

Fairfield KM. Vitamin supplementation in disease prevention. Seres D, ed. Waltham, MA: UpToDate. http://www.uptodate.com. Accessed December 7, 2018: 2020.

National Center for Complementary and Integrative Health, National Institutes of Health. Vitamins and Minerals. https://nccih.nih.gov/health/vitamins. Accessed: July 31, 2020.

Anti-Oxidants

Lifespan: Why We Age—and Why We Don't Have To by David Sinclair and Matthew LaPlante, Atria Books; Illustrated edition 2019

Macpherson H, Pipingas A, Pase MP. Multivitamin-multimineral supplementation and mortality: a meta-analysis of randomized controlled trials. Am J Clin Nutr. 2013 Feb;97(2):437-44. doi: 10.3945/ajcn.112.049304. Epub 2012 Dec 19. PMID: 23255568.

Sesso HD, Christen WG, Bubes V, Smith JP, MacFadyen J, Schvartz M, Manson JE, Glynn RJ, Buring JE, Gaziano JM. Multivitamins in the prevention of cardiovascular disease in men: the Physicians' Health Study II randomized controlled trial. JAMA. 2012 Nov 7;308(17):1751-60. doi: 10.1001/jama.2012.14805. PMID: 23117775; PMCID: PMC3501249.

Bjelakovic G, Nikolova D, Gluud LL, Simonetti RG, Gluud C. Mortality in randomized trials of antioxidant supplements for primary and secondary prevention: systematic review and meta-analysis. JAMA. 2007 Feb 28;297(8):842-57. doi: 10.1001/jama.297.8.842. Erratum in: JAMA. 2008 Feb 20;299(7):765-6. PMID: 17327526.

Fiber

Park Y, Subar AF, Hollenbeck A, Schatzkin A. Dietary fiber intake and mortality in the NIH-AARP diet and health study. Arch Intern Med. 2011 Jun 27;171(12):1061-8. doi: 10.1001/archinternmed.2011.18. Epub 2011 Feb 14. PMID: 21321288; PMCID: PMC3513325.

Yang J, Wang HP, Zhou L, Xu CF. Effect of dietary fiber on constipation: a meta analysis. World J Gastroenterol. 2012 Dec 28;18(48):7378-83. doi: 10.3748/wjg.v18.i48.7378. PMID: 23326148; PMCID: PMC3544045.

Probiotics

Dale HF, Rasmussen SH, Asiller ÖÖ, Lied GA. Probiotics in Irritable Bowel Syndrome: An Up-to-Date Systematic Review. Nutrients. 2019 Sep 2;11(9):2048. doi: 10.3390/nu11092048. PMID: 31480656; PMCID:PMC6769995.

Gut Crisis: How Diet, Probiotics, and Friendly Bacteria Help You Lose Weight and Heal Your Body and Mind by Robert Keith Wallace, PhD, Samantha Wallace, Dharma Publications, 2017

The Rest And Repair Diet: Heal Your Gut, Improve Your Physical and

Mental Health, and Lose Weight by Robert Keith Wallace, PhD, Samantha Wallace, Andrew Sternberg, MA Jim Davis, DO, and Alexis Farley, Dharma Publications, 2019

Metformin

Mohammed I, Hollenberg MD, Ding H, Triggle CR. A Critical Review of the Evidence That Metformin Is a Putative Anti-Aging Drug That Enhances Healthspan and Extends Lifespan. Front Endocrinol (Lausanne). 2021 Aug 5;12:718942. doi: 10.3389/fendo.2021.718942. PMID: 34421827; PMCID: PMC8374068.

Lifespan: Why We Age—and Why We Don't Have To by David Sinclair and Mathew LaPlante, ⬛Atria Books; Illustrated edition 2019

Green Tea

Pervin M, Unno K, Takagaki A, Isemura M, Nakamura Y. Function of Green Tea Catechins in the Brain: Epigallocatechin Gallate and its Metabolites. Int J Mol Sci. 2019 Jul 25;20(15):3630. doi: 10.3390/ijms20153630. PMID: 31349535; PMCID: PMC6696481.

Omega-3s

DiNicolantonio JJ, O'Keefe JH. The Importance of Marine Omega-3s for Brain Development and the Prevention and Treatment of Behavior, Mood, and Other Brain Disorders. Nutrients. 2020 Aug 4;12(8):2333. doi: 10.3390/nu12082333. PMID: 32759851; PMCID: PMC7468918.

Bischoff-Ferrari HA, Vellas B, Rizzoli R, Kressig RW, da Silva JAP, Blauth M, Felson DT, McCloskey EV, Watzl B, Hofbauer LC, Felsenberg D, Willett WC, Dawson-Hughes B, Manson JE, Siebert U, Theiler R, Staehelin HB, de Godoi Rezende Costa Molino C, Chocano-Bedoya PO, Abderhalden LA, Egli A, Kanis JA, Orav EJ; DO-HEALTH Research Group. Effect of Vitamin D Supplementation, Omega-3 Fatty Acid Supplementation, or a Strength-Training Exercise Program on Clinical Outcomes in Older Adults: The DO-HEALTH Randomized Clinical Trial. JAMA. 2020 Nov 10;324(18):1855-1868. doi: 10.1001/jama.2020.16909. PMID: 33170239; PMCID: PMC7656284.

Rauch, B.; Schiele, R.; Schneider, S.; Diller, F.; Victor, N.; Gohlke, H.; Gottwik, M.; Steinbeck, G.; Del Castillo, U.; Sack, R.; et al. OMEGA, a randomized, placebo-controlled trial to test the effect of highly purified omega-3 fatty acids on top of modern guideline-adjusted therapy after myocardial infarction. Circulation 2010, 122, 2152–2159.

McCarty, M.F.; DiNicolantonio, J.J.; Lavie, C.J.; O'Keefe, J.H. Omega-3 and prostate cancer: Examining the pertinent evidence. Mayo Clin. Proc. 2014, 89, 444–450.

DiNicolantonio, J.J.; Mccarty, M.F.; Lavie, C.J.; O'Keefe, J.H. Do omega-3 fatty acids cause prostate cancer? MO Med. 2013,110, 293–294.

Hu Y, Hu FB, Manson JE. Marine Omega-3 Supplementation and Cardiovascular Disease: An Updated Meta-Analysis of 13 Randomized Controlled Trials Involving 127 477 Participants. J Am Heart Assoc. 2019 Oct;8(19):e013543. doi: 10.1161/JAHA.119.013543. Epub 2019 Sep 30. PMID: 31567003; PMCID: PMC6806028.

Curcumin

Tomeh MA, Hadianamrei R, Zhao X. A Review of Curcumin and Its Derivatives as Anticancer Agents. Int J Mol Sci. 2019 Feb 27;20(5):1033. doi: 10.3390/ijms20051033. PMID: 30818786; PMCID: PMC6429287.

Salehi B, Stojanović-Radić Z, Matejić J, Sharifi-Rad M, Anil Kumar NV, Martins N, Sharifi-Rad J. The therapeutic potential of curcumin: A review of clinical trials. Eur J Med Chem. 2019 Feb 1;163:527-545. doi: 10.1016/j.ejmech.2018.12.016. Epub 2018 Dec 7. PMID: 30553144.

Lang A, Salomon N, Wu JC, Kopylov U, Lahat A, HarNoy O, et al. Curcumin in combination with mesalamine induces remission in patients with mild to moderate ulcerative colitis in a randomized controlled trial. Clin Gastroenterol Hepatol 2015;13:14449.e1.

Sudheeran SP, Jacob D, Mulakal JN, Nair GG, Maliakel A, Maliakel B, et al. Safety, tolerance, and enhanced efficacy of a bioavailable formulation of curcumin with fenugreek dietary fiber on occupational stress: a randomized, doubleblind, placebocontrolled pilot study. J Clin Psychopharmacol 2016;36:23643.

Aggarwal BB, Harikumar KB. Potential therapeutic effects of curcumin, the anti-inflammatory agent, against neurodegenerative, cardiovascular, pulmonary, metabolic, autoimmune and neoplastic Int J Biochem Cell Biol 2009;41:4059.

Venigalla M, Sonego S, Gyengesi E, Sharman MJ, Münch G. Novel promising therapeutics against chronic neuroinflammation and neurodegeneration in Alzheimer's disease. Neurochem Int 2016;95:6374.

Nelson KM, Dahlin JL, Bisson J, Graham J, Pauli GF, Walters MA. The Essential Medicinal Chemistry of Curcumin. J Med Chem. 2017 Mar 9;60(5):1620-1637. doi: 10.1021/acs.jmedchem.6b00975. Epub 2017 Jan 11. PMID: 28074653; PMCID: PMC5346970.

Resveratrol

Li J, Zhang CX, Liu YM, Chen KL, Chen G. A comparative study of anti-aging properties and mechanism: resveratrol and caloric restriction. Oncotarget. 2017 Aug 9;8(39):65717-65729. doi: 10.18632/oncotarget.20084. PMID: 29029466; PMCID: PMC5630366.

Lifespan: Why We Age—and Why We Don't Have To by David Sinclair and Matthew LaPlante, Atria Books; Illustrated edition 2019

Quercetin

Panche AN, Diwan AD, Chandra SR. Flavonoids: an overview. J Nutr Sci. 2016 Dec 29;5:e47. doi: 10.1017/jns.2016.41. PMID: 28620474; PMCID: PMC5465813.

Boots AW, Haenen GR, Bast A. Health effects of quercetin: from antioxidant to nutraceutical. Eur J Pharmacol. 2008 May 13;585(2-3):325-37. doi: 10.1016/j.ejphar.2008.03.008. Epub 2008 Mar 18. PMID: 18417116.

Bischoff SC. Quercetin: potentials in the prevention and therapy of disease. Curr Opin Clin Nutr Metab Care. 2008 Nov;11(6):733-40. doi: 10.1097/MCO.0b013e32831394b8. PMID: 18827577.

Lifespan: Why We Age—and Why We Don't Have To by David Sinclair and Matthew LaPlante, Atria Books; Illustrated edition 2019

Rapamycin

Blagosklonny MV. Rapamycin for longevity: opinion article. *Aging*

(Albany NY). 2019;11(19):8048-8067. doi:10.18632/aging.102355

Lifespan: Why We Age—and Why We Don't Have To by David Sinclair and Matthew LaPlante, Atria Books; Illustrated edition 2019

Fisetin

Yousefzadeh MJ, Zhu Y, McGowan SJ, Angelini L, Fuhrmann-Stroissnigg H, Xu M, Ling YY, Melos KI, Pirtskhalava T, Inman CL, McGuckian C, Wade EA, Kato JI, Grassi D, Wentworth M, Burd CE, Arriaga EA, Ladiges WL, Tchkonia T, Kirkland JL, Robbins PD, Niedernhofer LJ. Fisetin is a senotherapeutic that extends health and lifespan. EBioMedicine. 2018 Oct;36:18-28. doi: 10.1016/j.ebiom.2018.09.015. Epub 2018 Sep 29. PMID: 30279143; PMCID: PMC6197652.

Das J, Singh R, Ladol S, Nayak SK, Sharma D. Fisetin prevents the aging-associated decline in relative spectral power of α, β and linked MUA in the cortex and behavioral alterations. Exp Gerontol. 2020 Sep;138:111006. doi: 10.1016/j.exger.2020.111006. Epub 2020 Jun 24. PMID: 32592831.

Kashyap D, Garg VK, Tuli HS, Yerer MB, Sak K, Sharma AK, Kumar M, Aggarwal V, Sandhu SS. Fisetin and Quercetin: Promising Flavonoids with Chemopreventive Potential. Biomolecules. 2019 May 6;9(5):174. doi: 10.3390/biom9050174. PMID: 31064104; PMCID: PMC6572624.

NAD

Lifespan: Why We Age—and Why We Don't Have To by David Sinclair and Matthew LaPlante, Atria Books; Illustrated edition 2019

Martens CR, Denman BA, Mazzo MR, Armstrong ML, Reisdorph N, McQueen MB, Chonchol M, Seals DR. Chronic nicotinamide riboside supplementation is well-tolerated and elevates NAD+ in healthy middle-aged and older adults. Nat Commun. 2018 Mar 29;9(1):1286. doi: 10.1038/s41467-018-03421-7. PMID: 29599478; PMCID: PMC5876407.

Dollerup OL, Trammell SAJ, Hartmann B, Holst JJ, Christensen B, Møller N, Gillum MP, Treebak JT, Jessen N. Effects of Nicotinamide Riboside on Endocrine Pancreatic Function and Incretin Hormones in Nondiabetic Men With Obesity. J Clin Endocrinol Metab. 2019 Nov

1;104(11):5703-5714. doi: 10.1210/jc.2019-01081. PMID: 31390002

Wang K, Liu H, Hu Q, Wang L, Liu J, Zheng Z, Zhang W, Ren J, Zhu F, Liu GH. Epigenetic regulation of aging: implications for interventions of aging and diseases. Signal Transduct Target Ther. 2022 Nov 7;7(1):374. doi: 10.1038/s41392-022-01211-8. PMID: 36336680; PMCID: PMC9637765.

Coenzyme Q10

Pravst I, Rodríguez Aguilera JC, Cortes Rodriguez AB, Jazbar J, Locatelli I, Hristov H, Žmitek K. Comparative Bioavailability of Different Coenzyme Q10 Formulations in Healthy Elderly Individuals. Nutrients. 2020 Mar 16;12(3):784. doi: 10.3390/nu12030784. PMID: 32188111; PMCID: PMC7146408.

Amrit Kalash

Penza M, Montani C, Jeremic M, Mazzoleni G, Hsiao WL, Marra M, Sharma H, Di Lorenzo D. MAK-4 and -5 supplemented diet inhibits liver carcinogenesis in mice. BMC Complement Altern Med. 2007 Jun 8;7:19. doi: 10.1186/1472-6882-7-19. PMID: 17559639; PMCID: PMC1894988.

Dwivedi C, Agrawal P, Natarajan K, Sharma H. Antioxidant and protective effects of Amrit Nectar tablets on adriamycin- and cisplatin-induced toxicities. J Altern Complement Med. 2005 Feb;11(1):143-8. doi: 10.1089/acm.2005.11.143. PMID: 15750373.

Inaba R, Mirbod SM, Sugiura H. Effects of Maharishi Amrit Kalash 5 as an Ayurvedic herbal food supplement on immune functions in aged mice. BMC Complement Altern Med. 2005 Mar 25;5:8. doi: 10.1186/1472-6882-5-8. PMID: 15790423; PMCID: PMC1084244.

Vohra BP, Sharma SP, Kansal VK. Effect of Maharishi Amrit Kalash on age dependent variations in mitochondrial antioxidant enzymes, lipid peroxidation and mitochondrial population in different regions of the central nervous system of guinea-pigs. Drug Metabol Drug Interact. 2001;18(1):57-68. doi: 10.1515/dmdi.2001.18.1.57. PMID: 11522125.

Sharma H, Wallace RK. Ayurveda and Epigenetics. Medicina (Kaunas). 2020 Dec 11;56(12):687. doi: 10.3390/medicina56120687. PMID:

33322263; PMCID: PMC7763202.

Inaba R, Mirbod SM, Sugiura H. Effects of Maharishi Amrit Kalash 5 as an Ayurvedic herbal food supplement on immune functions in aged mice. BMC Complement Altern Med. 2005 Mar 25;5:8. doi: 10.1186/1472-6882-5-8. PMID: 15790423; PMCID: PMC1084244.

Triphala

Peterson CT, Denniston K, Chopra D. Therapeutic Uses of Triphala in Ayurvedic Medicine. J Altern Complement Med. 2017 Aug;23(8):607-614. doi: 10.1089/acm.2017.0083. Epub 2017 Jul 11. PMID: 28696777; PMCID: PMC5567597.

Baliga MS, et al. Scientific validation of the ethnomedicinal properties of the Ayurvedic drug Triphala: A review. Chin J Integr Med 2012;18:946–954

Ashwagandha

Speers AB, Cabey KA, Soumyanath A, Wright KM. Effects of *Withania somnifera* (Ashwagandha) on Stress and the Stress-Related Neuropsychiatric Disorders Anxiety, Depression, and Insomnia. Curr Neuropharmacol. 2021;19(9):1468-1495. doi: 10.2174/1570159X1966621071215 1556. PMID: 34254920; PMCID: PMC8762185.

Brahmi

Nemetchek MD, Stierle AA, Stierle DB, Lurie DI. The Ayurvedic plant Bacopa monnieri inhibits inflammatory pathways in the brain. J Ethnopharmacol. 2017 Feb 2;197:92-100. doi: 10.1016/j.jep.2016.07.073. Epub 2016 Jul 26. PMID: 27473605; PMCID: PMC5269610

Williams R, Münch G, Gyengesi E, Bennett L. Bacopa monnieri (L.) exerts anti-inflammatory effects on cells of the innate immune system in vitro. Food Funct. 2014 Mar;5(3):517-20. doi: 10.1039/c3fo60467e. PMID: 24452710.

Stough C, Lloyd J, Clarke J, Downey LA, Hutchison CW, Rodgers T, Nathan PJ. The chronic effects of an extract of Bacopa monniera (Brahmi) on cognitive function in healthy human subjects. Psychopharmacology (Berl). 2001 Aug;156(4):481-4. doi: 10.1007/s002130100815. Erratum in: Psychopharmacology (Berl). 2015 Jul;232(13):2427. Dosage error in article text. PMID: 11498727.

Peth-Nui T, Wattanathorn J, Muchimapura S, Tong-Un T, Piyavhatkul N, Rangseekajee P, Ingkaninan K, Vittaya-Areekul S. Effects of 12-Week Bacopa monnieri Consumption on Attention, Cognitive Processing, Working Memory, and Functions of Both Cholinergic and Monoaminergic Systems in Healthy Elderly Volunteers. Evid Based Complement Alternat Med. 2012;2012:606424. doi: 10.1155/2012/606424. Epub 2012 Dec 18. PMID: 23320031; PMCID: PMC3537209.

Rai D, Bhatia G, Palit G, Pal R, Singh S, Singh HK. Adaptogenic effect of Bacopa monniera (Brahmi). Pharmacol Biochem Behav. 2003 Jul;75(4):823-30. doi: 10.1016/s0091-3057(03)00156-4. PMID: 12957224.

Benson S, Downey LA, Stough C, Wetherell M, Zangara A, Scholey A. An acute, double-blind, placebo-controlled cross-over study of 320 mg and 640 mg doses of Bacopa monnieri (CDRI 08) on multitasking stress reactivity and mood. Phytother Res. 2014 Apr;28(4):551-9. doi: 10.1002/ptr.5029. Epub 2013 Jun 21. PMID: 23788517.

Calabrese C, Gregory WL, Leo M, Kraemer D, Bone K, Oken B. Effects of a standardized Bacopa monnieri extract on cognitive performance, anxiety, and depression in the elderly: a randomized, double-blind, placebo-controlled trial. J Altern Complement Med. 2008 Jul;14(6):707-13. doi: 10.1089/acm.2008.0018. PMID: 18611150; PMCID: PMC3153866.

Biohack #6

Gut Crisis: How Diet, Probiotics, and Friendly Bacteria Help You Lose Weight and Heal Your Body and Mind by Robert Keith Wallace, PhD, Samantha Wallace, Dharma Publications, 2017

The Rest And Repair Diet: Heal Your Gut, Improve Your Physical and Mental Health, and Lose Weight by Robert Keith Wallace, PhD, Samantha Wallace, Andrew Sternberg, MA Jim Davis, DO, and Alexis Farley, Dharma Publications, 2019

Puchalska P, Crawford PA. Multi-dimensional Roles of Ketone Bodies in Fuel Metabolism, Signaling, and Therapeutics. Cell Metab. 2017 Feb 7;25(2):262-284. doi: 10.1016/j.cmet.2016.12.022. PMID: 28178565; PM-CID: PMC5313038.

Miriam, B et al. Added Sugars and Cardiovascular Disease Risk in Children: A Scientific Statement From the American Heart Association, Circulation. 2017 May 09; 135(19): e1017–e1034

Serena, G et al. The Role of Gluten in Celiac Disease and Type 1 Diabetes. Nutrients 2015 Aug 26;7(9):7143-62

Leonardi, GC et al., Ageing: from inflammation to cancer. Immunity and Ageing 2018; 15:1Fasano, A, Intestinal permeability and its regulation by zonulin: diagnosis and therapeutic implications. Clinical Gastroenterology and Hepatology 2012; 10,1096-100

Fasano, A. Zonulin, Regulation of tight junctions, and autoimmune diseases. Annals of the New York Academy of Sciences 2012; 1258(1):25-33

Wallace, R.K. Ayurgenomics and Modern Medicine. Medicina 2020, 56, 661

Wallace, RK. The Microbiome in Health and Disease from the Perspective of Modern Medicine and Ayurveda. Medicina 2020; 56, 462.

Biohack #7

Gut Crisis: How Diet, Probiotics, and Friendly Bacteria Help You Lose Weight and Heal Your Body and Mind by Robert Keith Wallace, PhD, Samantha Wallace, Dharma Publications, 2017

The Rest And Repair Diet: Heal Your Gut, Improve Your Physical and Mental Health, and Lose Weigh by Robert Keith Wallace, PhD, Samantha Wallace, Andrew Sternberg, MA Jim Davis, DO, and Alexis Farley, Dharma Publications, 2019

Wallace, RK. The Microbiome in Health and Disease from the Perspective of Modern Medicine and Ayurveda. Medicina 2020; 56, 462.

Wallace, R.K. Ayurgenomics and Modern Medicine. Medicina 2020, 56, 661.

Biohack #8

Lee DH, Rezende LFM, Joh HK, Keum N, Ferrari G, Rey-Lopez JP, Rimm EB, Tabung FK, Giovannucci EL. Long-Term Leisure-Time Physical Activity Intensity and All-Cause and Cause-Specific Mortality: A Prospective Cohort of US Adults. Circulation. 2022 Aug 16;146(7):523-534. doi: 10.1161/CIRCULATIONAHA.121.058162. Epub 2022 Jul 25. PMID: 35876019; PMCID: PMC9378548.

Mu X, Liu S, Fu M, Luo M, Ding D, Chen L, Yu K. Associations of physical activity intensity with incident cardiovascular diseases and mortality among 366,566 UK adults. Int J Behav Nutr Phys Act. 2022 Dec 13;19(1):151. doi: 10.1186/s12966-022-01393-y. PMID: 36514169; PMCID: PMC9745930.

Wang Y, Nie J, Ferrari G, Rey-Lopez JP, Rezende LFM. Association of Physical Activity Intensity With Mortality: A National Cohort Study of 403 681 US Adults. JAMA Intern Med. 2021 Feb 1;181(2):203-211. doi: 10.1001/jamainternmed.2020.6331. PMID: 33226432; PMCID: PMC7684516.

Sanders LMJ, Hortobágyi T, Karssemeijer EGA, Van der Zee EA, Scherder EJA, van Heuvelen MJG. Effects of low- and high-intensity physical exercise on physical and cognitive function in older persons with dementia: a randomized controlled trial. Alzheimers Res Ther. 2020 Mar 19;12(1):28. doi: 10.1186/s13195-020-00597-3. PMID: 32192537; PMCID: PMC7082953.

Aguib Y, Al Suwaidi J. The Copenhagen City Heart Study (Østerbroundersøgelsen). Glob Cardiol Sci Pract. 2015 Oct 9;2015(3):33. doi: 10.5339/gcsp.2015.33. PMID: 26779513; PMCID: PMC4625209.

Atakan MM, Li Y, Koşar ŞN, Turnagöl HH, Yan X. Evidence-Based Effects of High-Intensity Interval Training on Exercise Capacity and Health: A Review with Historical Perspective. Int J Environ Res Public Health. 2021 Jul 5;18(13):7201. doi: 10.3390/ijerph18137201. PMID: 34281138; PMCID: PMC8294064.

Booth, FW; Roberts, C.K; Laye, M.J. Lack of exercise is a major cause of chronic diseases. Compr. Physiol. 2012, 2, 1143–1211

Hallal, PC. Andersen, L.B.; Bull, F.C.; Guthold, R.; Haskell, W.; Ekelund, U. Global physical activity levels: Surveillance progress, pitfalls, and prospects. Lancet 2012, 380, 247–257.

Bull, FC; Al-Ansari, SS; Biddle, S; Borodulin, K; Buman, MP; Cardon, G.; Carty, C.; Chaput, JP.; Chastin, S.; Chou, R.; et al. World Health Organization 2020 guidelines on physical activity and sedentary behaviour. Br. J. Sports Med. 2020, 54, 1451–1462.

Paluch AE, Gabriel KP, Fulton JE, et al. Steps per Day and All-Cause Mortality in Middle-aged Adults in the Coronary Artery Risk Development in Young Adults Study. *JAMA Netw Open.* 2021;4(9):e2124516. doi:10.1001/jamanetworkopen.2021.24516

Sleiman SF, Henry J, Al-Haddad R, El Hayek L, Abou Haidar E, Stringer T, Ulja D, Karuppagounder SS, Holson EB, Ratan RR, Ninan I, Chao MV. Exercise promotes the expression of brain derived neurotrophic factor (BDNF) through the action of the ketone body β-hydroxybutyrate. Elife. 2016 Jun 2;5:e15092. doi: 10.7554/eLife.15092. PMID: 27253067; PMCID: PMC4915811.

Cooney GM, et al. Exercise for depression. JAMA. 2014;311:2432.

Peterson DM. The benefits and risks of exercise. https://www.uptodate.com/contents/search. Accessed Sept. 15, 2017.

Greer TL, et al. Improvements in psychosocial functioning and health-related quality of life following exercise augmentation in patients with treatment response but nonremitted major depressive disorder: Results from the TREAD study. Depression and Anxiety. 2016;33:870.

Schuch FB, et al. Exercise as treatment for depression: A meta-analysis adjusting for publication bias. Journal of Psychiatric Research. 2016;77:42.

Zschucke E, et al. Exercise and physical activity in mental disorders: Clinical and experimental evidence. Journal of Preventive Medicine and Public Health. 2013;46:512.

Anderson E, et al. Effects of exercise and physical activity on anxiety. Frontiers in Psychiatry. 2013;4:1.

Isaac AR, Lima-Filho RAS, Lourenco MV. How does the skeletal muscle communicate with the brain in health and disease? Neuropharmacology. 2021 Oct 1;197:108744. doi: 10.1016/j.neuropharm.2021.108744. Epub 2021 Aug 5. PMID: 34363812

Saeed SA, Cunningham K, Bloch RM. Depression and Anxiety

Disorders: Benefits of Exercise, Yoga, and Meditation. Am Fam Physician. 2019 May 15;99(10):620-627. PMID: 31083878.

Wang WL, Chen KH, Pan YC, Yang SN, Chan YY. The effect of yoga on sleep quality and insomnia in women with sleep problems: a systematic review and meta-analysis. BMC Psychiatry. 2020 May 1;20(1):195. doi: 10.1186/s12888-020-02566-4. PMID: 32357858; PMCID: PMC7193366.

Groessl EJ, Liu L, Chang DG, Wetherell JL, Bormann JE, Atkinson JH, Baxi S, Schmalzl L. Yoga for Military Veterans with Chronic Low Back Pain: A Randomized Clinical Trial. Am J Prev Med. 2017 Nov;53(5):599-608. doi: 10.1016/j.amepre.2017.05.019. Epub 2017 Jul 20. PMID: 28735778; PMCID: PMC6399016.

Biohack #9

Arendt J. Melatonin: Countering Chaotic Time Cues. Front Endocrinol (Lausanne). 2019 Jul 16;10:391. doi: 10.3389/fendo.2019.00391. PMID: 31379733; PMCID: PMC6646716.

Poza JJ, Pujol M, Ortega-Albás JJ, Romero O; Insomnia Study Group of the Spanish Sleep Society (SES). Melatonin in sleep disorders. Neurologia (Engl Ed). 2022 Sep;37(7):575-585. doi: 10.1016/j.nrleng.2018.08.004. Epub 2020 Sep 18. PMID: 36064286.

Bueno APR, Savi FM, Alves IA, Bandeira VAC. Regulatory aspects and evidences of melatonin use for sleep disorders and insomnia: an integrative review. Arq Neuropsiquiatr. 2021 Aug;79(8):732-742. doi: 10.1590/0004-282X-ANP-2020-0379. PMID: 34550191.

Besag FMC, Vasey MJ, Lao KSJ, Wong ICK. Adverse Events Associated with Melatonin for the Treatment of Primary or Secondary Sleep Disorders: A Systematic Review. CNS Drugs. 2019 Dec;33(12):1167-1186. doi: 10.1007/s40263-019-00680-w. PMID: 31722088.

Reiter RJ, Ma Q, Sharma R. Melatonin in Mitochondria: Mitigating Clear and Present Dangers. Physiology (Bethesda). 2020 Mar 1;35(2):86-95. doi: 10.1152/physiol.00034.2019. PMID: 32024428.

Melhuish Beaupre LM, Brown GM, Gonçalves VF, Kennedy JL. Melatonin's neuroprotective role in mitochondria and its potential as a biomarker in aging, cognition and psychiatric disorders. Transl Psychiatry. 2021 Jun 2;11(1):339.

Li T, Jiang S, Han M, Yang Z, Lv J, Deng C, Reiter RJ, Yang Y. Exogenous melatonin as a treatment for secondary sleep disorders: A systematic review and meta-analysis. Front Neuroendocrinol. 2019 Jan;52:22-28. doi: 10.1016/j.yfrne.2018.06.004. Epub 2018 Jun 15. PMID: 29908879.

Foley HM, Steel AE. Adverse events associated with oral administration of melatonin: A critical systematic review of clinical evidence. Complement Ther Med. 2019 Feb;42:65-81. doi: 10.1016/j.ctim.2018.11.003. Epub 2018 Nov 3. PMID: 30670284.

Scholtens RM, van Munster BC, van Kempen MF, de Rooij SE. Physiological melatonin levels in healthy older people: A systematic review. J Psychosom Res. 2016 Jul;86:20-7. doi: 10.1016/j.jpsychores.2016.05.005. Epub 2016 May 10. PMID: 27302542.

Culpepper L, Wingertzahn MA. Over-the-Counter Agents for the Treatment of Occasional Disturbed Sleep or Transient Insomnia: A Systematic Review of Efficacy and Safety. Prim Care Companion CNS Disord. 2015 Dec 31;17(6):10.4088/PCC.15r01798. doi: 10.4088/PCC.15r01798. PMID: 27057416; PMCID: PMC4805417.

Zare Elmi HK, Gholami M, Saki M, Ebrahimzadeh F. Efficacy of Valerian Extract on Sleep Quality after Coronary Artery bypass Graft Surgery: A Triple-Blind Randomized Controlled Trial. Chin J Integr Med. 2021 Jan;27(1):7-15. doi: 10.1007/s11655-020-2727-1. Epub 2021 Jan 8. PMID: 33420602.

Murray BJ, Cowen PJ, Sharpley AL. The effect of Li 1370, extract of Ginkgo biloba, on REM sleep in humans. Pharmacopsychiatry. 2001 Jul;34(4):155-7. doi: 10.1055/s-2001-15876. PMID: 11518478.

Djokic G, Vojvodić P, Korcok D, Agic A, Rankovic A, Djordjevic V, Vojvodic A, Vlaskovic-Jovicevic T, Peric-Hajzler Z, Matovic D, Vojvodic J, Sijan G, Wollina U, Tirant M, Thuong NV, Fioranelli M, Lotti T. The Effects of Magnesium - Melatonin - Vit B Complex Supplementation in Treatment of Insomnia. Open Access Maced J Med Sci. 2019 Aug 30;7(18):3101-3105. doi: 10.3889/oamjms.2019.771. PMID: 31850132; PMCID: PMC6910806.

Sutanto CN, Loh WW, Kim JE. The impact of tryptophan

supplementation on sleep quality: a systematic review, meta-analysis, and meta-regression. Nutr Rev. 2022 Jan 10;80(2):306-316. doi: 10.1093/nutrit/nuab027. PMID: 33942088.

Dasdelen MF, Er S, Kaplan B, Celik S, Beker MC, Orhan C, Tuzcu M, Sahin N, Mamedova H, Sylla S, Komorowski J, Ojalvo SP, Sahin K, Kilic E. A Novel Theanine Complex, Mg-L-Theanine Improves Sleep Quality via Regulating Brain Electrochemical Activity. Front Nutr. 2022 Apr 5;9:874254. doi: 10.3389/fnut.2022.874254. PMID: 35449538; PMCID: PMC9017334.

Fetveit A, Skjerve A, Bjorvatn B. Bright light treatment improves sleep in institutionalised elderly-an open trial. Int J Geriatr Psychiatry. 2003 Jun;18(6):520-6. doi: 10.1002/gps.852. PMID: 12789673.

Higuchi S, Motohashi Y, Liu Y, Maeda A. Effects of playing a computer game using a bright display on presleep physiological variables, sleep latency, slow wave sleep and REM sleep. J Sleep Res. 2005 Sep;14(3):267-73. doi: 10.1111/j.1365-2869.2005.00463.x. PMID: 16120101.

Kanda K, Tochihara Y, Ohnaka T. Bathing before sleep in the young and in the elderly. Eur J Appl Physiol Occup Physiol. 1999 Jul;80(2):71-5. doi: 10.1007/s004210050560. PMID: 10408315.

Youngstedt SD, Kripke DF, Elliott JA. Is sleep disturbed by vigorous late-night exercise? Med Sci Sports Exerc. 1999 Jun;31(6):864-9. doi: 10.1097/00005768-199906000-00015. PMID: 10378914.

Biohack #10

The Brain Maker: The Power of Gut Microbes to Heal and Protect Your Brain for Life by Dr. David Perlmutter, Little, Brown Spark, 2015

Living in Balance with Maharishi AyurVeda by Robert Keith Wallace, PhD, Karin Pirc, MD, Julia Clarke, MS, MIU Press, 2023, in press

Schneider, RH, et al., Health Promotion with a Traditional System of Natural Health Care: Maharishi Ayurveda, 1990, Journal of Social Behavior and Personality, 5(3): 1-27

Waldschutz, R. Physiological and Psychological Changes Associated with Ayurvedic Purification Treatment, 1988, Erfahrungsheilkunde—Acta

Medico Empirica—Zeitschrift fur die drztliche Praxis, 2: 720-729

Herron RE, Fagan JB. Lipophil-mediated reduction of toxicants in humans: an evaluation of an ayurvedic detoxification procedure. Altern Ther Health Med. 2002 Sep-Oct;8(5):40-51. PMID: 12233802.

Biohack #11

Allada R, Bass J. Circadian Mechanisms in Medicine. N Engl J Med. 2021 Feb 11;384(6):550-561. doi: 10.1056/NEJMra1802337. PMID: 33567194; PMCID: PMC8108270.

Cornelissen G, Otsuka K. Chronobiology of Aging: A Mini-Review. Gerontology. 2017;63(2):118-128. doi: 10.1159/000450945. Epub 2016 Oct 22. PMID: 27771728.

Biohack #12

Tainio M, Jovanovic Andersen Z, Nieuwenhuijsen MJ, Hu L, de Nazelle A, An R, Garcia LMT, Goenka S, Zapata-Diomedi B, Bull F, Sá TH. Air pollution, physical activity and health: A mapping review of the evidence. Environ Int. 2021 Feb;147:105954. doi: 10.1016/j.envint.2020.105954. Epub 2020 Dec 19. PMID: 33352412; PMCID: PMC7816214.

Srinivasan TM. Pranayama and brain correlates. Anc Sci Life. 1991 Jul;11(1-2):2-6. PMID: 22556548; PMCID: PMC3336588.

Stancák A Jr, Pfeffer D, Hrudová L, Sovka P, Dostálek C. Electroencephalographic correlates of paced breathing. Neuroreport. 1993 Jun;4(6):723-6. doi: 10.1097/00001756-199306000-00031. PMID: 8347815.

Brennan SE, McDonald S, Murano M, McKenzie JE. Effectiveness of aromatherapy for prevention or treatment of disease, medical or preclinical conditions, and injury: protocol for a systematic review and meta-analysis. Syst Rev. 2022 Jul 26;11(1):148. doi: 10.1186/s13643-022-02015-1. PMID: 35883155; PMCID: PMC9317467.

Biohack #13

Bondy SC, Campbell A. Water Quality and Brain Function. Int J Environ Res Public Health. 2017 Dec 21;15(1):2. doi: 10.3390/ijerph15010002. PMID: 29267198; PMCID: PMC5800103.

Esperland D, de Weerd L, Mercer JB. Health effects of voluntary exposure to cold water: a continuing subject of debate. Int J Circumpolar Health. 2022 Dec;81(1):2111789. doi: 10.1080/22423982.2022.2111789. PMID: 36137565; PMCID: PMC9518606.

Lorenzo I, Serra-Prat M, Yébenes JC. The Role of Water Homeostasis in Muscle Function and Frailty: A Review. Nutrients. 2019 Aug 9;11(8):1857. doi: 10.3390/nu11081857. PMID: 31405072; PMCID: PMC6723611.

Biohack #14

Alexander R, Aragón OR, Bookwala J, Cherbuin N, Gatt JM, Kahrilas IJ, Kästner N, Lawrence A, Lowe L, Morrison RG, Mueller SC, Nusslock R, Papadelis C, Polnaszek KL, Helene Richter S, Silton RL, Styliadis C. The neuroscience of positive emotions and affect: Implications for cultivating happiness and wellbeing. Neurosci Biobehav Rev. 2021 Feb;121:220-249. doi: 10.1016/j.neubiorev.2020.12.002. Epub 2020 Dec 8. PMID: 33307046.

An HY, Chen W, Wang CW, Yang HF, Huang WT, Fan SY. The Relationships between Physical Activity and Life Satisfaction and Happiness among Young, Middle-Aged, and Older Adults. Int J Environ Res Public Health. 2020 Jul 4;17(13):4817. doi: 10.3390/ijerph17134817. PMID: 32635457; PMCID: PMC7369812.

Steptoe A, Deaton A, Stone AA. Subjective wellbeing, health, and ageing. Lancet. 2015 Feb 14;385(9968):640-648. doi: 10.1016/S0140-6736(13)61489-0. Epub 2014 Nov 6. PMID: 25468152; PMCID: PMC4339610.

Dharma Parenting: Understand Your Child's Brilliant Brain for Greater Happiness, Health, Success, and Fulfillment by Robert Keith Wallace, PhD, and Frederick Travis, PhD, Tarcher/Perigree, 2016

Biohack #15

Palacios J, Eichholtz P, Kok N. Moving to productivity: The benefits of healthy buildings. PLoS One. 2020 Aug 6;15(8):e0236029. doi: 10.1371/journal.pone.0236029. PMID: 32760082; PMCID: PMC7410200.

The Coherence Effect: Tapping into the Laws of Nature that Govern Health, Happiness, and Higher Brain Functioning by Robert Keith Wallace, PhD, Jay B. Marcus, and Chris S. Clark, MD, Armin Lear Press, 2020

The Neurophysiology of Enlightenment: How the Transcendental Meditation and TM-Sidhi Program Transform the Functioning of the Human Body by Robert Keith Wallace, PhD, Dharma Publications, 2016

Hagelin JS, et al. Effects of group practice of the Transcendental Meditation program on preventing violent crime in Washington, DC: results of the National Demonstration Project, June-July 1993. Social Indicators Research 47: 153-201, 1999

Orme-Johnson DW, et al. International peace project in the Middle East: The effect of the Maharishi Technology of the Unified Field. Journal of Conflict Resolution 32: 776–812, 1988

Orme-Johnson DW, et al. The long-term effects of the Maharishi Technology of the Unified Field on the quality of life in the United States (1960 to 1983). Social Science Perspectives Journal 2:127-146, 1988

Orme-Johnson DW, et al. Preventing terrorism and international conflict: Effects of large assemblies of participants in the Transcendental Meditation and TM-Sidhi programs. Journal of Offender Rehabilitation 36: 283–302, 2003

Brown CL. Overcoming barriers to use of promising research among elite Middle East policy groups. Journal of Social Behavior and Personality 17:489-546, 2005

Cavanaugh KL. Time series analysis of U.S. and Canadian inflation and unemployment: A test of a field-theoretic hypothesis. Proceedings of the American Statistical Association, Business and Economics Statistics Section (Alexandria, VA: American Statistical Association): 799–804, 1987

Cavanaugh KL, King KD. Simultaneous transfer function analysis of

Okun's misery index: Improvements in the economic quality of life through Maharishi's Vedic Science and technology of consciousness. Proceedings of the American Statistical Association, Business and Economics Statistics Section (Alexandria, VA: American Statistical Association): 491–496, 1988

Davies JL. Alleviating political violence through enhancing coherence in collective consciousness. Dissertation Abstracts International 49(8): 2381A, 1989

Gelderloos P, et al. The dynamics of US–Soviet relations, 1979–1986: Effects of reducing social stress through the Transcendental Meditation and TM-Sidhi program. Proceedings of the Social Statistics Section of the American Statistical Association (Alexandria, VA: American Statistical Association): 297–302, 1990

Dillbeck MC. Test of a field theory of consciousness and social change: Time series analysis of participation in the TM-Sidhi program and reduction of violent death in the U.S. Social Indicators Research 22: 399–418, 1990

Assimakis PD, Dillbeck MC. Time series analysis of improved quality of life in Canada: Social change, collective consciousness, and the TM-Sidhi program. Psychological Reports 76: 1171–1193, 1995

Hatchard GD, et al. A model for social improvement. Time series analysis of a phase transition to reduced crime in Merseyside metropolitan area. Psychology, Crime, and Law 2: 165–174, 1996

Dillbeck MC, et al. The Transcendental Meditation program and crime rate change in a sample of forty-eight cities. Journal of Crime and Justice 4: 25–45, 1981

Dillbeck MC, et al. Test of a field model of consciousness and social change: The Transcendental Meditation and TM-Sidhi program and decreased urban crime. The Journal of Mind and Behavior 9: 457–486, 1988

Dillbeck MC. et al. Consciousness as a field: The Transcendental Meditation and TM-Sidhi program and changes in social indicators. The Journal of Mind and Behavior 8: 67–104, 1987.

Biohack #16

Sherman R, Hickner J. Academic physicians use placebos in clinical practice and believe in the mind-body connection. J Gen Intern Med. 2008 Jan;23(1):7-10. doi: 10.1007/s11606-007-0332-z. Epub 2007 Nov 10. PMID: 17994270; PMCID: PMC2173915.

Ortega Á, Salazar J, Galban N, Rojas M, Ariza D, Chávez-Castillo M, Nava M, Riaño-Garzón ME, Díaz-Camargo EA, Medina-Ortiz O, Bermúdez V. Psycho-Neuro-Endocrine-Immunological Basis of the Placebo Effect: Potential Applications beyond Pain Therapy. Int J Mol Sci. 2022 Apr 11;23(8):4196. doi: 10.3390/ijms23084196. PMID: 35457014; PMCID: PMC9028312.

Tavel M.E. The Placebo Effect: The Good, the Bad, and the Ugly. Am. J. Med. 2014;127:484–488. doi: 10.1016/j.amjmed.2014.02.002.

Wager T.D., Atlas L.Y. The Neuroscience of Placebo Effects: Connecting Context, Learning and Health. Nat. Rev. Neurosci. 2015;16:403–418. doi: 10.1038/nrn3976

Bernstein MH, Brown WA. The placebo effect in psychiatric practice. Curr Psychiatr. 2017 Nov;16(11):29-34. PMID: 29910696; PMCID: PMC6003660.

Zion SR, Crum AJ. Mindsets Matter: A New Framework for Harnessing the Placebo Effect in Modern Medicine. Int Rev Neurobiol. 2018;138:137-160. doi: 10.1016/bs.irn.2018.02.002. Epub 2018 Mar 20. PMID: 29681322.

Crum AJ, Langer EJ. Mind-set matters: exercise and the placebo effect. Psychol Sci. 2007 Feb;18(2):165-71. doi: 10.1111/j.1467-9280.2007.01867.x. PMID: 17425538.

Human Physiology: Expression of Veda and the Vedic Literature 4th Edition by Dr. Tony Nader, MD, PhD, Maharishi Vedic University; 2001

Ramanyan in Human Physiology, by Dr. Tony Nader, MD, PhD, Maharishi Vedic University; 4th edition, 2001

One Unbounded Ocean of Consciousness: Simple Answers to Big Questions in Life by Dr. Tony Nader, MD, PhD, Penguin Random House Grupo Editorial, 2021

The Hero with a Thousand Faces by Joseph Campbell, New World

Library; Third edition, 2008

Estebsari F, Dastoorpoor M, Khalifehkandi ZR, Nouri A, Mostafaei D, Hosseini M, Esmaeili R, Aghababaeian H. The Concept of Successful Aging: A Review Article. Curr Aging Sci. 2020;13(1):4-10. doi: 10.2174/1874609812666191023130117. PMID: 31657693; PMCID: PMC7403646.

Science of Being and Art of Living: Transcendental Meditation by Maharishi Mahesh Yogi, MUM Press, Kindle edition, 2011

Maharishi Mahesh Yogi on the Bhagavad-Gita, A New Translation and Commentary, Chapters 1-6, MUM Press, 2016

The Supreme Awakening: Experiences of Enlightenment Throughout Time –And How You Can Cultivate Them by Craig Pearson, MIU Press, 2013

Index

A

B

C

D

Printed in the USA
CPSIA information can be obtained
at www.ICGtesting.com
LVHW041954020124
767833LV00010B/304